PREPARING FOR THE FUTURE OF HIV/AIDS IN AFRICA

A SHARED RESPONSIBILITY

Committee on Envisioning a Strategy to Prepare for the
Long-Term Burden of HIV/AIDS: African Needs and U.S. Interests

Board on Global Health

INSTITUTE OF MEDICINE
OF THE NATIONAL ACADEMIES

THE NATIONAL ACADEMIES PRESS
Washington, D.C.
www.nap.edu

THE NATIONAL ACADEMIES PRESS 500 Fifth Street, N.W. Washington, DC 20001

This study was supported by grants and contributions to the National Academy of Sciences from the Atlantic Philanthropies (Grant 3852); BD (Becton, Dickinson and Company) (Contribution 6387); the Bill & Melinda Gates Foundation (Grant 6445); the Carnegie Corporation of New York (Grant 6179); the Doris Duke Charitable Foundation (Grant 6143); the Ford Foundation (Grant 8407); the Institute of International Education (Grant 6456); Johnson & Johnson Services, Inc. (Grant 6346); Merck & Co., Inc. (Grant 6552); and Pfizer, Inc. (Grant 6336). The study also received in-kind support from the Rockefeller Foundation. Any opinions, findings, conclusions, or recommendations expressed in this publication are those of the author(s) and do not necessarily reflect the view of the organizations or agencies that provided support for this project.

International Standard Book Number-13: 978-0-309-16018-6
International Standard Book Number-10: 0-309-16018-9

Additional copies of this report are available from the National Academies Press, 500 Fifth Street, N.W., Lockbox 285, Washington, DC 20055; (800) 624-6242 or (202) 334-3313 (in the Washington metropolitan area); Internet, http://www.nap.edu.

For more information about the Institute of Medicine, visit the IOM home page at: **www.iom.edu.**

Printed in the United States of America

The serpent has been a symbol of long life, healing, and knowledge among almost all cultures and religions since the beginning of recorded history. The serpent adopted as a logotype by the Institute of Medicine is a relief carving from ancient Greece, now held by the Staatliche Museen in Berlin.

Suggested citation: IOM (Institute of Medicine). 2011. *Preparing for the Future of HIV/ AIDS in Africa: A Shared Responsibility.* Washington, DC: The National Academies Press.

"Knowing is not enough; we must apply.
Willing is not enough; we must do."
—Goethe

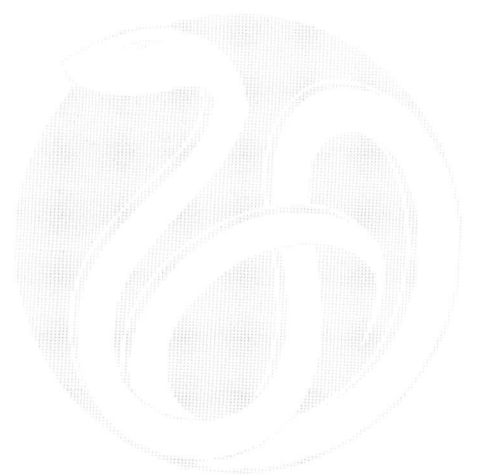

INSTITUTE OF MEDICINE
OF THE NATIONAL ACADEMIES

Advising the Nation. Improving Health.

THE NATIONAL ACADEMIES
Advisers to the Nation on Science, Engineering, and Medicine

The **National Academy of Sciences** is a private, nonprofit, self-perpetuating society of distinguished scholars engaged in scientific and engineering research, dedicated to the furtherance of science and technology and to their use for the general welfare. Upon the authority of the charter granted to it by the Congress in 1863, the Academy has a mandate that requires it to advise the federal government on scientific and technical matters. Dr. Ralph J. Cicerone is president of the National Academy of Sciences.

The **National Academy of Engineering** was established in 1964, under the charter of the National Academy of Sciences, as a parallel organization of outstanding engineers. It is autonomous in its administration and in the selection of its members, sharing with the National Academy of Sciences the responsibility for advising the federal government. The National Academy of Engineering also sponsors engineering programs aimed at meeting national needs, encourages education and research, and recognizes the superior achievements of engineers. Dr. Charles M. Vest is president of the National Academy of Engineering.

The **Institute of Medicine** was established in 1970 by the National Academy of Sciences to secure the services of eminent members of appropriate professions in the examination of policy matters pertaining to the health of the public. The Institute acts under the responsibility given to the National Academy of Sciences by its congressional charter to be an adviser to the federal government and, upon its own initiative, to identify issues of medical care, research, and education. Dr. Harvey V. Fineberg is president of the Institute of Medicine.

The **National Research Council** was organized by the National Academy of Sciences in 1916 to associate the broad community of science and technology with the Academy's purposes of furthering knowledge and advising the federal government. Functioning in accordance with general policies determined by the Academy, the Council has become the principal operating agency of both the National Academy of Sciences and the National Academy of Engineering in providing services to the government, the public, and the scientific and engineering communities. The Council is administered jointly by both Academies and the Institute of Medicine. Dr. Ralph J. Cicerone and Dr. Charles M. Vest are chair and vice chair, respectively, of the National Research Council.

www.national-academies.org

Consultants

ROBERT BLACK, Chairman, Department of International Health; Edgar Berman Professor in International Health; Director, Institute for International Programs, Johns Hopkins University, Bloomberg School of Public Health, Baltimore, MD

LAWRENCE GOSTIN, Linda D. and Timothy J. O'Neill Professor of Global Health Law, Georgetown University Law Center, Washington, DC

MARIA MERRITT, Assistant Professor, Department of International Health, Johns Hopkins University, Bloomberg School of Public Health and Berman Institute of Bioethics, Baltimore, MD

Staff

ELIZABETH HAYTMANEK, Program Officer
PATRICIA CUFF, Senior Program Officer
KATHLEEN OSTAPKOVICH, Research Associate (until August 2010)
KENISHA PETERS, Research Assistant
RACHEL PITTLUCK, Intern
JULIE WILTSHIRE, Financial Associate
PATRICK KELLEY, Director, Boards on Global Health and African Science Academy Development

Editor

RONA BRIERE

Reviewers

This report has been reviewed in draft form by individuals chosen for their diverse perspectives and technical expertise, in accordance with procedures approved by the National Research Council's Report Review Committee. The purpose of this independent review is to provide candid and critical comments that will assist the institution in making its published report as sound as possible and to ensure that the report meets institutional standards for objectivity, evidence, and responsiveness to the study charge. The review comments and draft manuscript remain confidential to protect the integrity of the deliberative process. We wish to thank the following individuals for their review of this report:

Victor De Gruttola, Harvard University, Department of Biostatistics
Mark Dybul, Georgetown University, O'Neill Institute for National and Global Health Law
Jason Farley, School of Nursing, Department of Community Public Health Nursing, Johns Hopkins University; Faculty of Health Sciences, Division of Nursing, Stellenbosch University
Barry Kistnasamy, National Institute for Occupational Health, South Africa
Jimmy Kolker, UNICEF
Joseph-Matthew Mfutso-Bengo, University of Malawi, College of Medicine
Marjorie Opuni-Akuamoa, Johns Hopkins University, Bloomberg School of Public Health, Department of International Health
Doreen Ramogola-Masire, Botswana-UPenn Partnership, Botswana
Eleanor Ross, University of Witwatersrand, Department of Social Work, School of Human and Community Development

Susan Scrimshaw, The Sage Colleges
Sten Vermund, Vanderbilt University
Alan Whiteside, University of KwaZulu-Natal
Catherine Wilfert, Elizabeth Glaser Pediatrics AIDS Foundation
Ajume Wingo, University of Colorado at Boulder, Philosophy Department

Although the reviewers listed above have provided many constructive comments and suggestions, they were not asked to endorse the conclusions or recommendations nor did they see the final draft of the report before its release. The review of this report was overseen by **Ronald Brookmeyer,** Professor, Department of Biostatistics, School of Public Health, University of California, Los Angeles; and **William Holzemer,** Dean and Professor, College of Nursing-Newark & New Brunswick, Rutgers, The State University of New Jersey. Appointed by the National Research Council and the Institute of Medicine, they were responsible for making certain that an independent examination of this report was carried out in accordance with institutional procedures and that all review comments were carefully considered. Responsibility for the final content of this report rests entirely with the authoring committee and the institution.

Acknowledgments

This report is a product of the cooperation and contributions of many people. The committee would like to thank all the speakers and moderators who participated in committee meetings and workshops, as well as others who provided information, input, and assistance. They include Patti Abbott, Lori Bollinger, Sue K. Brown, Elizabeth Bukusi, Kathy Cahill, Robin Crewe, Rosanne Diab, Robert Einterz, Robert Garris, Jenni Gillies, Eric Goosby, Wilfred Griekspoor, James Hakim, Mark Heywood, Joan Holloway, Leigh Johnson, Michael Johnson, Quarraisha Karim, Sylvester Kimaiyo, Surabhi Lal, Umesh Lalloo, Princeton Lyman, Morakeng Malatji, Stephen Mallinga, Leslie Mancuso, Joana Mangueira, Xola Mati, Tony Mbewu, Phakamile Truth Mngadi, Steve Morrison, Mbalawa Mugabe, Neal Nathanson, Laura Podio, Takalani Rambau, Danni Ramduth, Celicia Serenata, Darrell Singer, Papa Salif Sow, Devi Sridhar, Ruth Stark, Jeff Sturchio, Nthabiseng Taole, Leana Uys, Brian Williams, and David Wilson.

This report would have not been possible without the generous financial contributions of the study's sponsors: the Atlantic Philanthropies; BD (Becton, Dickinson and Company); the Bill & Melinda Gates Foundation; the Carnegie Corporation of New York; the Doris Duke Charitable Foundation; the Ford Foundation; the Institute of International Education; Johnson & Johnson Services, Inc.; Merck & Co., Inc; and Pfizer, Inc. The study also received in-kind support from the Rockefeller Foundation.

Contents

xi

Summary

In many African[1] countries, where the burden of HIV/AIDS is the greatest in the world, the number of new infections is growing more rapidly than the availability of treatment. Unless this trend is reversed, HIV/AIDS can be expected to continue at a high rate of transmission for many decades to come. Despite the recent mobilization of donor funds, resources are strained, and the capacity of the region's health care systems to absorb the increasing treatment load is precarious. Ensuring adequate institutional and human resources to meet the challenges of HIV/AIDS in Africa 10 to 15 years into the future will therefore require visionary strategic planning and investments in capacity building.

In this context, the Institute of Medicine (IOM) tasked a committee of experts to recommend affordable, sustainable strategies that both African nations and the United States can implement to address the long-term burden of HIV/AIDS.[2] The committee concluded that the burden of morbidity and mortality in Africa cannot be alleviated through treatment alone. Treatment can reach only a fraction of those who need it, and its costs are unsustainable. Therefore, greater emphasis must be placed on preventing new infections.

---

[1] For purposes of brevity, unless otherwise noted, the term *Africa* denotes sub-Saharan Africa throughout the report.

[2] The statement of task for this study did not call for, nor was the committee constituted to develop a social, behavioral, or biomedical science research agenda for addressing HIV/AIDS. The committee recognizes that advances in these areas could radically change the future of the epidemic.

THE BURDEN OF HIV/AIDS

In 2009, approximately 33.3 million people globally were living with HIV; an estimated 2 million people died as a result of HIV/AIDS; and 2.6 million people, including 370,000 children, were newly infected (UNAIDS, 2010). Of those global HIV infections, 22.5 million were in Africa; this figure represents 68 percent of the global total, while the number of newly infected in the region represents 69 percent of the global total (UNAIDS, 2010). According to the World Health Organization's (WHO's) most recent guidelines, just 36 percent of those needing treatment are receiving it (WHO, 2010). Moreover, the committee's projections indicate that the need for treatment will increase dramatically over the next decade.

In addition to its toll on individuals and households, HIV/AIDS has had devastating impacts on four key sectors of African society: development, health, the state, and academia. The burden of the epidemic has compromised the achievement of key Millennium Development Goals in Africa and has led to declines in the growth of total gross domestic product (GDP) in the most affected countries.

KEY FINDINGS AND CONCLUSIONS

Local Responses to Global Solutions

Although countries in Africa share many similarities, they also differ greatly in culture, history, politics, and education. As such, it is not surprising to find that HIV epidemics across Africa range from highly concentrated to highly generalized, and the responses by African nations have been equally varied, ranging from intense interventions to complete denial of HIV disease. Given this heterogeneity, as well as the diversity of African institutions and circumstances, the programs and policies recommended in this report require tailoring to local circumstances. The committee was not constituted to recommend specific actions for particular African countries; rather, in keeping with the theme of shared responsibility, the committee recommends approaches for African countries that can be adapted to their needs and priorities.

The Future Impact of Current Decisions

In 2020, the morbidity, mortality, and resource and financial burdens faced by the U.S. government and African countries for the ensuing decades will depend on decisions made today:

- Currently, people are becoming in need of treatment more rapidly than they are being placed on treatment. Therefore, although the death rate from AIDS has fallen, deaths among those in need of treatment will continue. There are two ways of closing the treatment gap: increase treatment coverage, and reduce incidence. The incidence (i.e., number of new cases) of HIV infection must be reduced before the burdens of treatment and mortality can begin to decline.

- Because treatment is a form of prevention, delaying initiation of treatment once it is recommended for an individual will also delay the realization of reduced need for treatment. If earlier treatment is expanded, of course, many more people will need to be on treatment in the short term. Moreover, the decline in numbers requiring treatment will be gradual, so that any reduction in incidence achieved in 2010 will only partially reduce the burden of HIV/AIDS by 2020. Thus the benefits of reduced incidence need to be considered over a period of decades.
- The burden of HIV/AIDS is extremely sensitive to alternative policies. The course of the epidemic, costs, and the lives of millions of individuals will be affected by decisions made today regarding, for example, early versus late treatment initiation, coverage with second-line versus first-line regimens, program quality versus quantity, and investment in treatment versus prevention.

Implications of the Projected HIV/AIDS Burden in Africa for U.S. Interests

With the launch of the U.S. President's Emergency Plan for AIDS Relief (PEPFAR) in 2003, the United States established itself as a global leader in expanding care and treatment in the fight against HIV/AIDS in Africa. Through PEPFAR and support for the Global Fund to Fight AIDS, Tuberculosis and Malaria, the United States helped galvanize an extraordinary global response to a single disease and mobilize donor and private-sector resources on an unprecedented scale. Despite this momentum, the expected expansion of the epidemic in the coming decade portends significant challenges for the United States and the global community in sustaining these commitments.

In the United States, the effects of a historic global financial crisis and a domestic deficit approaching $2 trillion will likely drive greater congressional scrutiny of spending on foreign assistance. Ironically, moreover, the success of the U.S. HIV/AIDS effort has increased attention to other African health challenges, which may drive competition in resource allocation among health priorities. Beyond health, the scope of U.S. development assistance in Africa has expanded dramatically in the last decade to include food security, climate change, and unemployment. As the United States seeks new forms of engagement in Africa that provide greater political and economic leverage than traditional development and humanitarian assistance, options are reduced because the commitment to support Africans on life-saving antiretroviral therapy (ART) cannot be withdrawn to advance diplomatic goals.

As new HIV infections continue to outstrip the world's ability to provide

ART to those in need, the costs of treatment alone will consume ever larger proportions of available resources. The combination of competing health and development demands, the rising cost burden of HIV/AIDS treatment, and continued resource constraints will force difficult choices for U.S. policy makers. As the largest single contributor to global HIV/AIDS resource flows to date, the United States will need to manage these choices in a way that does not compromise the global achievements in HIV/AIDS, advances U.S. interests, and strengthens global capacities to respond to HIV/AIDS and other global health challenges.

One way for the United States to accomplish these goals while addressing its own fiscal concerns is to transition to a model for long-term sustainability based on shared responsibility with African partner states and the broader international community. By looking to African partners to assume increasing responsibility for leadership, management, and investment of resources in HIV/AIDS, the United States would be promoting a future of self-reliance and self-sustainability in the region. Under this shared-responsibility model, the United States would assist African partner states in developing the leadership, academic, medical, research, and other capacities necessary to assume that responsibility effectively. Countries with demonstrated political will, an emphasis on prevention, and efficient, transparent health management would receive stronger financial commitments with less oversight or intervention from the United States. Implementation of this model would necessitate greater accountability and transparency in the investments being made by each African partner state. The United States would need to set ambitious but realistic objectives for the next 10 to 15 years and place an urgent and consistent focus on prevention of new HIV infections.

Strategies to Build Capacity for Prevention, Treatment, and Care of HIV/AIDS in Africa, 2020–2025

A major requirement if African states are to assume greater responsibility for responding to their HIV/AIDS epidemics is to strengthen health care systems in the region by building institutional and human resource capacity. Successful capacity building supports national health plans and health care system development. Host country partners would take the lead, since government capacity is itself crucial to the future course of the African HIV/AIDS epidemic.

Strategies for Highly Affected Nations in Africa: Making the Most of Existing Capacities

Given increasing numbers of patients, shortages of trained medical personnel, and financial constraints, treatment must be provided more efficiently, as is encouraged by the Joint United Nations Programme on HIV/AIDS (UNAIDS) Treatment 2.0 platform. The committee has identified a number of strategies for making the most of existing African capacities.

First, scale-up of HIV/AIDS prevention, treatment, and care programs must rely not just on health care professionals but also on management and support staff from outside the clinical health sector who can free up time for health care providers to perform clinical work.

A second strategy—task sharing, in which physicians, nurses, dentists, and other health professionals delegate health care responsibilities and relevant knowledge to others, including community health workers—can make more efficient use of existing human resources and ease bottlenecks in service delivery. Sharing of responsibility may also involve the delegation of some clearly delineated tasks to newly created cadres of health workers who receive specific competency-based training.

Harnessing the expertise and building the capacity of the informal health care sector is a third viable strategy. Informal health workers, such as untrained family members or friends, merchants and shopkeepers, and traditional healers, are found in every health care system; the weaker the formal sector, the greater impact they have. Where formal health care facilities are not easily accessed, this group of informal health workers is the first and most important point of call for people in search of health care services.

A fourth strategy is to tap the potential of information and communication technology (ICT). Recent major advances have enabled applications such as teleconsultations, telereferrals, electronic patient records, and training of community health workers to support such aspects of health care as prevention, diagnosis, and patient management and care.

A fifth strategy entails planning the African health workforce on the basis of projected needs. To this end, African governments will need to establish, strengthen, and maintain health personnel information systems that collect, analyze, and translate data into effective health workforce policies and planning.

Existing African institutions also hold great potential for mitigating the future impact of the HIV/AIDS burden. In particular, partnerships and regional collaborations involving universities and other academic training programs in developing countries can be used to exchange technical assistance in HIV/AIDS prevention, treatment, and care through visits, training, and ongoing communication. African science academies can make important contributions to these efforts, providing balanced, multidisciplinary, authoritative, and evidence-based locally appropriate advice. Finally, coordinating core public health functions through national public health institutes and health resource partner institutions and networks can result in more efficient use of resources, improved delivery of public health services, and increased capacity to respond decisively to public health threats and opportunities.

Strategies for the United States: Supporting Partnerships and Other Capacity-Building Programs

The U.S. private sector, nongovernmental organizations, militaries, and academic institutions can help build capacity for HIV/AIDS prevention, treatment, and care by participating in partnerships with African institutions.

First, public–private partnerships can contribute to the fight against HIV/AIDS by enhancing the skills and capacities of local organizations; increasing the public sector's access to the expertise and core competencies of the private sector; facilitating the scale-up of proven, cost-effective interventions through private-sector networks and associations; expanding the reach of interventions by accessing target populations (for instance, through workplace programs); and sharing costs and promoting synergy among programs.

Second, faith-based organizations can make important contributions because they exist in cities, villages, and even the most rural regions of low-income countries, providing between 30 and 40 percent of health care services. Moreover, while governments and political climates change over time, communities of faith generally remain intact.

Third, military partnerships can support the strengthening of local health care systems by building the partners' capacity to provide needed services for HIV/AIDS. These services include behavioral interventions tailored to the risk factors faced by military personnel.

Finally, academic partnerships, including "twinning" between universities and technical and vocational schools, are yet another means of building capacity. In the context of this study, twinning is defined as a bilateral, mutually beneficial capacity-building partnership formed to mitigate the effects of HIV/AIDS. Parity is an essential feature of such a partnership; new skills, processes, and knowledge should be acquired by both partners through the process.

Strategies to Ensure an Ethical Decision-Making Capacity for HIV/AIDS Policy and Programming in Africa

Decisions about HIV/AIDS policy and programming are made at three levels. At the *macro* level, governments determine the overall health budget and its distribution across categories such as human resources, hospital operating expenses, research, and disease-specific treatment programs. At the *meso* level, institutions such as ministries of health, hospitals, and clinics determine which services they will provide and how much they will allocate for such expenses as staff, equipment, and supplies. At the *micro* level, health care providers decide what expenditures to recommend for the benefit of each individual patient. At any of these three levels of decision making, when people whose needs exceed available resources have approximately the same clinical status or risk exposure, medical criteria are insufficient to guide resource allocation decisions. From a moral point of view, then, the decision-making process for resource allocation must incorporate robust safeguards not only against discrimination but also against arbitrary or self-serving exercises of power.

One safeguard is to identify and empower stakeholders in particular settings who should have far more influence in such decision making than they actually do (such as patients and the general public). A complementary approach is to identify relatively enduring processes through which resource allocation decisions are made and to enhance the ethical capacity of those already empowered. The range of such actors might include local health service providers, local health care system managers, HIV/AIDS program implementers, civil society (community-based and nongovernmental organizations), traditional community leaders, local public officials, academic institutions, national public officials, regional organizations, and the media (to promote responsible and balanced reporting of information so as to foster participatory democracy).

The committee concluded that there is a need to build capacity for ethical decision making in Africa with respect to policies, programs, and resource allocation for HIV/AIDS in their populations. Core competencies for ethical decision making need to be defined in such areas as budgeting, management, evidence assessment, communications, and health policy analysis. Insufficient capacity may exist to deal with counterethical pressures from powerful actors. In many cases, government officials also need assistance in developing accountability and competence, particularly in priority setting and fair allocation of scarce resources.

RECOMMENDATIONS

The committee's recommendations are a first step toward exercising the shared responsibility of the United States and Africa to prepare for the future of HIV/AIDS. These recommendations are in three areas: the future impact of current decisions, implications of the projected burden of HIV/AIDS for the United States and Africa, and strategies to prepare for the long-term burden of the epidemic.

The Future Impact of Current Decisions

Recommendation 2-1[3]: *Measure incidence.* African countries, with the support of donors, should develop and implement cost-effective methods

---

[3] The committee's recommendations are numbered according to the chapters of the report in which they appear. Thus, for example, Recommendation 2-1 is the first recommendation in chapter 2.

for accurately measuring the level of and change in HIV/AIDS incidence to enable better planning and evaluation of HIV/AIDS prevention programs.[4]

Recommendation 2-2: *Analyze trade-offs.* The U.S. government should support countries in developing projections of the future burden of their HIV/AIDS epidemics and in assessing the implications of alternative national HIV/AIDS policies for human welfare, capacity, and resources so policy makers can make informed decisions on HIV/AIDS-related trade-offs.

Implications of the Projected Burden of HIV/AIDS for the United States and Africa

Recommendation 3-1[5]: *Emphasize a new contract approach that incentivizes shared responsibility.* The Office of the Global AIDS Coordinator should emphasize, develop, and implement a more binding, negotiated contract approach at the country level. The contract should incentivize shared responsibility whereby additive donor resources are provided to a large extent as matching funds for partner countries' investments of their own domestic resources in health. Such matching funds should not be a uniform ratio; rather, the ratio should vary based on each African partner's ability to contribute.

Recommendation 3-2: *Develop a U.S. roadmap for HIV/AIDS in 2020.* The White House and the Office of the Global AIDS Coordinator should develop a U.S. roadmap for HIV/AIDS in 2020 incorporating a model of U.S.–African shared responsibility that makes prevention a priority and balances bilateral and multilateral funding. The roadmap should:

- Give priority to prevention as a central tenet of a sustainable long-term response to the HIV/AIDS epidemic. To this end, steps should be taken to:
  - strengthen country-level surveillance and monitoring of the epidemic to ensure adequate and reliable data with which to estimate incidence rates (see Recommendation 2-1);
  - encourage the UNAIDS-recommended approach of targeted prevention strategies tailored to in-country priority populations, applying evidence-based public health approaches;

---

[4] As described in Chapter 2, laboratory-based assays for the calculation of incidence estimates are in development and are urgently needed to provide important epidemiological data on trends of the epidemic and the effectiveness of interventions so that limited resources can be directed most efficiently to limit the epidemic's further spread.

[5] See counterpart Recommendation 4-3 directed to African countries.

- increase access to and coverage of synergistic combinations of known effective prevention technologies; and
- expand research and investments in new prevention technologies.

- Strike an optimal balance between bilateral and multilateral mechanisms for HIV/AIDS funding. The United States should seek to capitalize on the strategic complementarity of bilateral and multilateral funding flows and engagement and work to strengthen multilateral institutions toward that end. U.S. policy makers should encourage greater involvement of emerging economic powers, including Brazil, China, Russia, and India, in international forums and activities on HIV/AIDS and in strengthening of South–South collaborations addressing the epidemic.[6]

Recommendation 3-3: *Integrate health and development.* Congress should support greater integration of U.S.-funded HIV/AIDS interventions with broader U.S. global health initiatives and African countries' comprehensive development plans. As Congress contemplates an overhaul of the U.S. Foreign Assistance Act, it should seek to encourage greater flexibility in development funding to ensure that assistance for both health and development meets recipient country priorities.

Recommendation 4-1: *Develop 10-year country roadmaps.* In parallel with the U.S. strategic planning called for in Recommendation 3-2, individual national HIV/AIDS coordinating bodies in Africa should develop, articulate, and update national 10-year roadmaps for combating HIV/AIDS. Each roadmap should take into account the implications of long-term projections of the national HIV/AIDS burden for institutions, communities, and resource requirements. As part of their roadmap, African governments should:

- invest sufficiently in HIV/AIDS prevention, following globally accepted best prevention practices;
- disclose national and subnational prevention outcomes and impacts and how they vary geographically and over time; and
- perform yearly evaluations to determine success as measured by change in HIV incidence data, as discussed in Recommendation 2-1.

Recommendation 4-2: *Develop and promote more efficient models of HIV/AIDS care and treatment.* African countries should invest in, evaluate, and

---

[6] South–South collaborations involve a horizontal relationship between two or more developing countries in which technical assistance in HIV/AIDS prevention, treatment, and care is exchanged through visits, training, and ongoing communication.

apply more efficient models of HIV/AIDS care and treatment and promote those models through South–South learning exchanges.

Recommendation 4-3[7]: *Establish a governance contract.* African countries should establish a negotiated contract with U.S. agencies that includes programmatic targets and delineates each partner's responsibilities and expectations within a shared-responsibility approach. African governments should fully maintain the role and function of leadership and stewardship for policies and program implementation in their countries' health sector.

Strategies to Prepare for the Long-Term Burden of the Epidemic

Recommendation 5-1: *Analyze and plan for meeting workforce requirements.* African governments and international organizations should assess and plan for meeting national workforce requirements for responding to the long-term burden of HIV/AIDS.

- **Recommendation 5-1a:** Through partnership programs and other investments, African governments and institutions, along with U.S. private companies, academic institutions, foundations, and civil society organizations, should establish national databases and information systems for health care worker statistics, as well as bolster the analytic capacity of national planners for determining human resource needs.
- **Recommendation 5-1b:** African governments and institutions should create staffing models to optimize the impact of the health care workforce. Such models should include developing cadres of managers and support staff outside the clinical health sector, encouraging needs-based training and task sharing within the health sector, focusing on retention through compensation and other incentives, utilizing information technologies, and harnessing the informal health sector.
- **Recommendation 5-1c:** In Africa, governments and institutions should work together in planning the African health care workforce based on projected needs derived from national data and analyses of future human resource requirements. Such planning should involve ministries of health, education, finance, public service, and labor. The private sector and the academic and medical communities should also be brought to the table for such national human resource planning exercises.

Recommendation 5-2: *Utilize existing African capacity.* African governments and international donors should recognize, invest in, strengthen, and

---

[7] See counterpart Recommendation 3-1 directed to the U.S. Office of the Global AIDS Coordinator.

utilize currently existing capacity within African institutions and networks to provide local solutions for responding to the HIV/AIDS epidemic. This capacity includes South–South and regional partnerships, universities, African science academies, national public health institutes, and other networks within Africa.

Recommendation 5-3: *Develop government leadership and management in health.* U.S. government agencies and programs, foundations, and academic institutions should invest in the development of African leadership and management in the health sector.

- **Recommendation 5-3a:** U.S. government agencies, such as the Health Resources and Service Administration (HRSA), the U.S. Agency for International Development (USAID), and the U.S. Centers for Disease Control and Prevention (CDC) and its global counterparts, should be actively engaged in leadership and management development, and the International Association of Public Health Institutes should be tapped as a resource for advancing these efforts.
- **Recommendation 5-3b:** U.S. foundations and academic institutions should invest in African leadership and management development through programs that educate African scientists and scholars who may then take on leadership positions in their own countries.

Recommendation 5-4: *Invest in innovative partnerships.* Private-sector organizations, professional organizations, faith-based organizations, academic and research institutions, militaries, foundations, and civil society organizations should increase funding for and participation in meaningful, effective, and innovative partnerships designed to build African capacity now to address the full extent of the HIV/AIDS burden over the next 10 years.

- **Recommendation 5-4a:** New U.S.–African partnerships between local vocational or technical schools that train allied health professionals, laboratory technicians, informatics specialists, and/or health administrators should be explored and encouraged.
- **Recommendation 5-4b:** Innovative North–South and South–South partnerships that build human resources for health should be developed. In North–South partnerships, African counterparts should take the lead in developing and controlling the partnership agenda.

Recommendation 6-1: *Enable and reinforce capacity for ethical decision making.* Donors and governments should help build capacity for ethical decision making by adequately funding education and training in the disciplines of ethics, human rights, and pertinent aspects of the law. This training should include both educational and implementation components.

Recommendation 6-2: *Donors and governments should support civil society organizations where they exist and help develop them in other places over time.* As a first step, the focus should be on procedural justice. Therefore, U.S. government agencies, including the State Department, USAID, and the Department of Health and Human Services, should provide technical and financial support to recipients of their health assistance for the establishment of effective mechanisms for procedural justice, including transparency, accountability, and responsibility.

Recommendation 6-3: *Professionals with training in ethics should be incorporated into multisectoral teams.* To increase the capacity for ethical decision making at the national level, professionals with training in ethics should be incorporated into national government multisectoral teams that include ministries of health, finance, and education, as well as other government ministries whose work is relevant to HIV/AIDS; civil society organizations; educational institutions; professional organizations; and nongovernmental organizations.

A CALL TO ACTION

Just as Africa is a mosaic of countries and cultures, HIV/AIDS is a mosaic of different epidemics in different countries and regions in Africa and around the world, each with its own dynamic character; the politics, economics, and sociocultural drivers of HIV/AIDS are distinct in different settings. As a result, programs and policies should reflect local circumstances. Therefore, the recommendations in this report will need to be tailored to individual countries and their epidemics.

Many of the recommendations imply a need to perform implementation and operations research[8]—as well as ongoing evaluation—of programs, partnerships, and interventions to combat HIV/AIDS in Africa. Such efforts can identify the optimal approaches for carrying out the recommendations in specific contexts. Moreover, no single strategy can meet the challenge of HIV/AIDS; countries will need to adopt multipronged strategies, tailored to local circumstances.

It is the committee's hope that this report will contribute to the global fight

---

[8] Operations research seeks to identify and address barriers related to the performance of specific projects. Implementation research seeks to create generalizable knowledge that can be applied across settings and contexts to answer central questions (such as how multiple interventions can be packaged effectively to capture cost efficiencies and reduce the splintering of health systems into disease-specific programs) (Madon et al., 2007).

against HIV/AIDS in Africa and beyond. This report focuses on Africa, where the incidence and prevalence of HIV/AIDS are the greatest in the world and where the impact of the pandemic is most pronounced in all sectors of society. Nonetheless, the committee's recommendations and the array of strategies identified in this report can and should be applied to the broader global context.

REFERENCES

Madon, T., K. J. Hofman, L. Kupfer, and R. I. Glass. 2007. Implementation science. *Science* 318(5857):1728-1729.

UNAIDS (The Joint United Nations Programme on HIV/AIDS). 2010. *Global report: UNAIDS report on the global AIDS epidemic 2010*. Geneva: UNAIDS.

WHO. 2010. *Towards universal access: Scaling up priority HIV/AIDS interventions in the health sector. Progress report 2010*. Geneva: WHO.

1

Introduction

The trajectory of the HIV/AIDS pandemic[1] over the next decade is expected to place demands on health care systems manyfold greater than have occurred to date. The global incidence and prevalence of HIV/AIDS and the natural progression of the disease is to the point where costly treatments are required, as well as the collateral effects on individuals, families, communities, and nations, have ominous implications for the future. The magnitude of the problem is most severe in Africa,[2] which accounted for 68 percent of all HIV-infected individuals and 69 percent of all new infections in 2009 (UNAIDS, 2010). The current burden of morbidity due to the pandemic is straining resources for prevention, treatment, and care; again, this strain is felt most acutely in Africa, where the capacity of health care systems to absorb at least a tenfold increase in treatment load is especially precarious.

Antiretroviral drugs have prolonged the life of a fraction of affected individuals, yet even this accomplishment has required immense effort, supported by multibillion-dollar investments by the Global Fund to Fight AIDS, Tuberculosis and Malaria, as well as the U.S. President's Emergency Plan for AIDS Relief (PEPFAR) and other sources of assistance. This effort is taxing human resource capacities at the risk of increasingly negative collateral effects on other health and development initiatives, especially in Africa. In fact, the impressive mobilization of donor funds to combat HIV/AIDS has created an environment in which

---

[1] A pandemic is an epidemic occurring worldwide or over a very wide area, crossing boundaries of several countries, and usually affecting a large number of people.

[2] For purposes of brevity, unless otherwise noted, the term *Africa* denotes sub-Saharan Africa throughout the report.

the shortage of human resources has replaced funding as the major obstacle to implementing national prevention, care, and treatment programs. Furthermore, the expected growth in the burden of HIV/AIDS in the coming decade portends significant challenges for the United States and the global community in sustaining and expanding commitments to combating HIV/AIDS in Africa.

STATEMENT OF TASK AND STUDY SCOPE

In this context, the task of the Institute of Medicine (IOM) Committee on Envisioning a Strategy to Prepare for the Long-Term Burden of HIV/AIDS: African Needs and U.S. Interests was to develop innovative strategies that can be used by the United States and other donor countries to respond to the challenge of HIV/AIDS in the coming decades through institutional and human resource capacity building (see Box 1-1).[3] This report is the product of that effort.

Although the committee's statement of task speaks to the global nature of HIV/AIDS, it was clear from the outset of the study that the focus would be on Africa, the region most affected and most challenged by the pandemic. Accordingly, half of the committee members are from African states. Moreover, as the committee undertook its deliberations, it quickly became apparent that time and resource constraints would necessitate confining the scope of the study to the African context. Even within Africa, however, the epidemic is heterogeneous, as described below.

Finally, with respect to its recommendations, the committee recognizes that the social determinants of health (the conditions in which people live and work, such as access to education, women's status, and poverty) are critically important, and that improvements in these areas would help mitigate the impacts of the global HIV/AIDS pandemic. In this report, however, the committee confines its recommendations to the domain of health care systems.

THE BURDEN OF HIV/AIDS

In 2009, approximately 33.3 million people globally were living with HIV; an estimated 2 million people died as a result of HIV/AIDS; and 2.6 million people, including 370,000 children, were newly infected (UNAIDS, 2010). Of those global HIV infections, 22.5 million were in Africa; as noted earlier, this figure represents 68 percent of the global total, while the number of newly infected represents 69 percent of the global total (UNAIDS, 2010). Expansion of the HIV/AIDS epidemic has varied across Africa. The regional variation in prevalence of HIV among those aged 15–49 is shown in Table 1-1. The countries

---

[3] The statement of task for this study did not call for, nor was the committee constituted to develop, a social, behavioral, or biomedical science research agenda for addressing HIV/AIDS. The committee recognizes that advances in these areas could radically change the future of the epidemic.

BOX 1-1
Statement of Task

The Institute of Medicine will convene an ad hoc committee to describe the long term trajectory for the global AIDS pandemic, why the problem is critically important to the U.S. and international interests and to highly affected countries, the relationship between current capacities and needed capacities, and provide consensus conclusions and recommendations for how the United States and other donor countries can innovatively respond to the challenge through institutional and human resource capacity building. Specific questions to be addressed are:

1. A decade from now (2018) what is the best projection for global incidence and burden of HIV/AIDS and its demographic and geographic distribution? What is the sensitivity of these projections to assumptions concerning the prevention of HIV infection?
2. What are the long term human resource and institutional implications of the projected global HIV infection prevalence on U.S. health, economic, diplomatic, industrial, scientific, academic, and other interests?
3. What are the implications of the projected HIV incidence and overall HIV/AIDS burden from the perspective of African governments and institutions including academia and the health care sector?
4. What should be the strategies for the U.S. and highly affected nations to develop now in order to ensure domestic and international capacities for highly effective HIV prevention, treatment, and care efforts in the 2018–2023 timeframe? What structures, systems, and professions would be necessary to implement these strategies?
   a. What could be the strategic role of U.S., African, and other universities in highly affected areas with respect to support for "twinning" at the level of individual faculty members, departments, schools, and entire universities?
   b. What could be the strategic role of other American institutions in supporting "twinning" for global capacity building relevant to HIV prevention, treatment, and care? What are the pro's and con's of these forms of assistance?
   c. How should South-South and regional considerations be incorporated into national plans?
   d. What should be the role of African science academies in supporting HIV/AIDS prevention, treatment, and care strategy refinements at the national level?
5. What are the implications of the projected HIV incidence and burden of HIV/AIDS for the capacity of resource-constrained countries to conduct decision making in an ethical manner?

TABLE 1-1 Prevalence Among Those Aged 15–49 in African Countries by sub-Saharan African Region

Country	Prevalence Among Those Aged 15–49 (%)
West Africa	
Ghana	1.8
Liberia	1.5
Senegal	0.9
Central Africa	
Chad	3.4
Congo	3.4
Central African Republic	4.7
Eastern Africa	
Kenya	6.3
Tanzania	5.6
Uganda	6.5
Southern Africa	
Botswana	24.8
South Africa	17.8
Zimbabwe	14.3

SOURCE: UNAIDS, 2010.

included in the table were chosen because they are representative of the HIV prevalence in their region.

In addition to the regional variation in prevalence, three main categories of countries are battling the HIV/AIDS epidemic in Africa. First are the hyperendemic countries of southern Africa. In addition to hosting the greatest burden of disease, these countries have faced their own particular issues because some of them are middle- or lower-middle-income countries, such as South Africa and Botswana, while others are extremely poor, such as Malawi and Zambia. Additionally, while South Africa bears a great burden of disease in terms of total numbers, Botswana, Lesotho, Namibia, and Swaziland struggle with enormous proportional burdens. The second category consists of low-income countries that bear a great burden of disease, such as Uganda, Ethiopia, Kenya, and Tanzania. These countries face a different set of challenges. While their epidemics may not be on the same scale as those in the highest-prevalence countries, their resources are much more limited. For them, the challenge is how to sustain treatment when the cost of ART is many times their per capita health expenditure. The third category comprises countries with low-prevalence epidemics, such as Angola and Senegal. It is important to keep this category separate from the other two as it may not be cost-effective for them to invest in HIV/AIDS prevention, treatment, and care with the same urgency as countries in the other two categories.

The committee distinguishes these three main categories of countries to make the point that HIV/AIDS is a mosaic of epidemics in Africa. As a result, the programs and policies recommended in this report will require tailoring to local circumstances; the type of epidemic and specific country context should inform the type and degree of response from African and U.S. governments and other stakeholders. Where African countries have the necessary financial resources, infrastructure, and political will, they are strongly encouraged to implement these recommendations with their own resources; financial support to these countries from the United States and other donor nations should be contingent on their using national resources to the extent possible. For the lowest-income, less-capable African countries with weak leadership around HIV/AIDS, the United States and other donors should play a larger role in the capacity-building aspects of the shared-responsibility paradigm, including leadership and infrastructure development, and should maintain strict oversight of their financial support. Given the projected burden of HIV/AIDS in the coming decades, support from international donors today can help build the infrastructure, political will, and institutional and human resource capacity that African nations will need to meet their own country-specific HIV/AIDS needs and priorities in 2020 and beyond. The committee did not deem it appropriate to prescribe certain recommendations for specific African countries; rather, in keeping with the theme of shared responsibility, it is the committee's hope that African countries will adapt the committee's recommendations to their own needs and priorities.

With respect to treatment, the percentage of those needing ART who were receiving it as of 2009 depends on which World Health Organization (WHO) guidelines are applied. According to the 2006 guidelines, treatment should be initiated at a CD4 cell count[4] below 200 cells/μL. By this criterion, just 53 percent of those needing ART were receiving it in Africa as of December 2009. The picture becomes bleaker, however, if the 2010 guidelines are applied, under which treatment should be initiated at a CD4 cell count of below 350 cells/μL. By this criterion, the percentage needing and receiving treatment in Africa drops to just 36 percent (WHO, 2010).

According to the committee's projections (see Figure 2-5 in Chapter 2), the need for treatment will increase manyfold over the next decade. By then, approximately 35 million people will be infected in Africa, and the estimated number on treatment will be 7 million, or a mere 60 percent of those needing treatment according to the 2006 WHO guidelines.

---

[4] CD4 cell count is the number of CD4 cells (T-helper lymphocytes with CD4 cell surface marker), used to assess immune status, susceptibility to opportunistic infections, and need for ART and opportunistic infection prophylaxis and to define AIDS (CD4 below 200).

ADDRESSING THE LONG-TERM BURDEN OF
HIV/AIDS: GUIDING PRINCIPLES

In deliberating about how best to address the long-term burden of HIV/AIDS in Africa, the committee was particularly mindful of several factors: (1) the projected trajectory of the epidemic (see Appendix A), (2) the resource and funding constraints facing the United States and other donor nations, (3) the limited resources and capacity of African states, (4) the need for sustainable approaches, and (5) the overarching imperative to lessen the suffering of those affected by HIV/AIDS. Two guiding principles emerged from consideration of these factors:

- The burden of morbidity and mortality in Africa cannot be alleviated through treatment interventions alone. Treatment can reach only a fraction of those who need it, and its costs are not sustainable for the foreseeable future. Therefore, greater emphasis must be placed on reducing incidence by preventing new infections.
- African states and societies must become full partners in the fight against HIV/AIDS. If this shared-responsibility model is to be feasible, however, they must have greater resources (particularly human resources) and capacity at all levels, from national governments to local communities.

STUDY APPROACH

In conducting this study, the 12-member committee drew on the extensive and varied experience of its members; testimony from subject matter experts in the field; input from numerous organizations; and the published literature on HIV/AIDS epidemiology and issues of financing, foreign policy, the global health workforce, and ethics related to the pandemic. Over the course of the study, the committee held four meetings and two public workshops. The first committee meeting, held in Washington, DC, in February 2010, featured the project sponsors and a discussion of the committee's charge; a portion of this meeting was open to the public and included testimony from U.S.-based experts in HIV/AIDS epidemiology, foreign policy, and programming. At the second committee meeting, held in Pretoria, South Africa, in April 2010, the committee heard from a range of African government officials, program managers, academics, and activists during a 2-day public workshop held in collaboration with the Academy of Science of South Africa. Through the generous sponsorship of the Rockefeller Foundation, the committee held its third meeting in June 2010 in Bellagio, Italy, to formulate its recommendations and draft this report. In September 2010, the committee held its fourth and final meeting in Washington, DC, to review a draft of the report and reach consensus on its recommendations. The information gathered from these many sources informed the committee's deliberations, the content of this report, and the committee's recommendations for how the U.S. and African governments and nongovernmental institutions should prepare for the future impacts of HIV/AIDS in Africa.

ORGANIZATION OF THE REPORT

Chapter 2 sets the stage for the remainder of the report by examining the future impact of current decisions with respect to the potential for reducing HIV/AIDS incidence and treatment needs, as well as the policy choices and associated trade-offs that must be considered in designing optimum strategies to combat the epidemic in Africa. Chapters 3 and 4, respectively, elaborate on the foundation for these decisions by detailing the implications of the burden of HIV/AIDS for the United States and African states and societies.

Chapter 5 builds on Chapters 2 through 4 to present strategies identified by the committee as both effective and feasible for responding to the long-term burden of HIV/AIDS in Africa. The emphasis of these strategies is on sustainability and shared responsibility between the United States and other donor nations and African states. Finally, Chapter 6 addresses the crucial issue of building the capacity of African leadership for ethical decision making in dealing with the very difficult and inevitable choices that must be made in the face of the gap between treatment needs and available resources. Chapters 2 through 6 end with recommendations formulated by the committee as a result of its deliberations on the respective topics.

In addition, four appendixes are provided. Appendix A addresses the issue of projecting the future burden of HIV/AIDS, examining both epidemiological and economic projections. Appendix B briefly reviews the demographic variation of the epidemic in Africa. Appendix C presents the agendas for the two public workshops held in conjunction with the committee's February and April 2010 meetings, while Appendix D contains biographical sketches of the committee members.

REFERENCES

UNAIDS (The Joint United Nations Programme on HIV/AIDS). 2010. *Global report: UNAIDS report on the global AIDS epidemic 2010.* Geneva: UNAIDS.

WHO. 2010. *Towards universal access: Scaling up priority HIV/AIDS interventions in the health sector. Progress report 2010.* Geneva: WHO.

2

The Future Impact of Current Decisions

Key Findings

- A number of prevention interventions, including prevention of mother-to-child transmission, male circumcision, a vaginal micro-bicide containing tenofovir, and high coverage of counseling and testing, hold promise for reducing HIV incidence.
- Treatment is a form of prevention; the earlier in the course of infection individuals are started on treatment, the sooner the preventive effects of treatment will be realized.
- Policy choices involve trade-offs in the areas of early versus late treatment initiation, coverage with second-line versus first-line regimens, and quality versus quantity of programs. The trade-off between investments in prevention versus treatment is largely spurious given their potential synergism.
- A plausible "best" scenario for 2020 projects the total number of patients on treatment to reach 7 million in Africa and the annual expenditures for treatment to total approximately $7 billion.
- Under several plausible scenarios, treatment costs will eventually decline as a proportion of the health budgets of African countries, enabling them to move toward greater ownership of their countries' prevention, treatment, and care objectives.

While policy makers' decisions can have only a small effect on the magnitude of the HIV/AIDS epidemic and its burden[1] by 2020, decision makers do have time to set a new course for the epidemic so that the prospects for 2020 onward look more optimistic than is the case today. Depending on decisions outlined in this chapter, morbidity, mortality, and resource and financial burdens faced in 2020 by the U.S. government and African countries for the ensuing decades could differ by a factor of 10 or more. Available policy choices include not only the rate at which HIV/AIDS treatment is scaled up, but also how it is scaled up and how scale-up is linked to the effectiveness of prevention. This chapter examines in turn the potential for reducing HIV incidence, the potential for reducing treatment need, and the key policy choices and associated trade-offs that decision makers must consider in formulating long-term strategies for responding to the epidemic.

POTENTIAL FOR REDUCING HIV INCIDENCE

As noted in Chapter 1, a guiding principle of this study is the need to reduce the incidence of HIV (defined as the number of new infections during a given period of time). The number of people needing treatment in the short term is driven mainly by those currently infected; over time, however, those acquiring infection will require treatment. Reductions in the incidence of HIV infection will take some time to alter the burdens of treatment and mortality but are necessary if these burdens are eventually to decline. Currently, people are becoming in need of treatment more rapidly than they are being placed on treatment. This means that, although the death rate from AIDS has fallen, deaths among those in need of treatment will continue. To improve this situation, two things must happen: treatment coverage must increase, and incidence must fall. The pattern of incidence of new HIV infections will determine the treatment need or, if treatment is not available, the death rate.

The ability to measure and monitor HIV incidence is critical to the capacity to monitor epidemiological trends within selected populations; assess the effectiveness of intervention programs; and appropriately direct limited resources for treatment, prevention, and care. Knowledge of HIV incidence is necessary both to understand transmission patterns and to project the burden of HIV infection in different demographic and at-risk populations. Reliable information on HIV incidence is especially important to support prevention programs in resource-

---

[1] The burden of HIV/AIDS for a population in a given year can be defined to include five components: its impact on health, on national income, on donor and domestic spending, on the workload of health care providers and institutions, and on the dependence of patients on a daily dose of medication for their survival. The committee's quantitative estimates of burden in this chapter and Appendix A focus on HIV prevalence as an indicator of the total health burden, on the total number of patients on treatment, on the total spending required to sustain treatment, and on spending as a share of projected national health expenditures. Chapter 4 considers in more depth the burden of HIV prevalence on the health sector in African states.

limited African countries that continue to bear a disproportionate share of the global burden of HIV/AIDS. Improved estimates of HIV incidence are essential for evaluating ongoing HIV/AIDS prevention and treatment programs in these settings and for guiding the most effective use of the billions of dollars that will be spent on combating the epidemic in the coming years (Busch et al., 2010; Fiamma et al., 2010; Mastro et al., 2010; Welte et al., 2010).

In the past, several methods, including prospective follow-up of cohorts of HIV-negative individuals and mathematical models based on epidemiological information about HIV prevalence and AIDS diagnoses or death rates, were used to estimate incidence over time. Unfortunately, these methods were subject to bias with respect to being unrepresentative of larger populations; were costly; and were directly impacted by the introduction of antiretroviral therapy (ART), which affected the calculation of incidence based on prevalence estimates. As a result of these complexities and limitations of epidemiological and modeling approaches to measuring HIV incidence, there has long been an effort to develop laboratory methods that can distinguish recent from established or long-term HIV infection as a means of estimating HIV incidence. Several assays and algorithms have been developed that have been partially successful in estimating incidence in cross-sectional surveys. However, there is an urgent need to make these assays more sensitive and specific so that accurate estimates of incidence will be available to medical and policy leaders.

Evidence of What Works from Randomized Controlled Trials

Experimental evidence on successful HIV prevention interventions is limited. The randomized controlled trial (RCT), which ensures internal validity in testing and intervention, relies on a clear, ethical, and replicable intervention that can be randomly allocated to a treatment and a control group (Susser, 1996). An effect will be more apparent when the effect size is large against a control providing no effect, and is more readily achieved for biomedical procedures for which adherence is ensured. In addition, the sample size is dependent upon the number of events that can be measured in the control arm. Such favorable conditions are not found when an intense, culturally specific intervention is appropriately implemented. Often because of a low incidence of HIV infection, intermediate behavioral endpoints have been used as surrogates for HIV incidence. However, the complex, context-specific relationship between risk behaviors and acquisition of HIV makes such intermediate endpoints inadequate without further validation. When HIV incidence has been used as an endpoint, many interventions have shown no effect (Padian et al., 2010).

Individual RCTs test the efficacy of interventions in preventing the acquisition of HIV in individuals. In such trials in the mid-1990s, prevention of mother-to-child transmission was confirmed as effective in reducing transmission to the baby by almost 70 percent (Connor et al., 1994). More recently, adult male circumcision has repeatedly been shown to reduce acquisition in men by 60 percent (Auvert et al., 2005; Bailey et al., 2007; Gray et al., 2007). Recently, hope for an effective vaccine has been raised by marginally significant results of a trial of a combined vaccine (Rerks-Ngarm et al., 2009). And further evidence of efficacy has been found for a vaginal microbicide containing tenofovir (Karim et al., 2010). While these results suggest the possibility of the eventual development of new prevention technologies, much work will be required before these early results can be translated into widely used products.

Moreover, the efficacy of an intervention in an individual does not imply its effect on the spread of HIV in a population. The population-level impact of an efficacious approach can be estimated through models or tested in community RCTs. Community RCTs make it possible to test interventions that can be implemented only at the population level (such as media campaigns) or programs that combine multiple approaches. They are often large and logistically complex, however, and therefore are few in number and provide little evidence of impact. See Box 2-1 for a summary of available results of such trials for sexually transmitted infections (STIs), a potential cofactor of HIV.

BOX 2-1
Results of Community Randomized Controlled Trials
of Interventions for Sexually Transmitted Infections

In Mwanza, Tanzania, syndromic management of STIs led to significantly (42 percent over 2 years) lower HIV incidence in intervention compared with control communities (Grosskurth et al., 1995). In Rakai, Uganda, mass antibiotic administration to control STIs and thereby HIV led to significant reductions in syphilis (relative risk [RR] = 0.8; 95 percent confidence interval [CI] 0.71–0.89) and trichomonas (RR = 0.59; 95 percent CI 0.38–0.91) but no reductions in gonorrhoea, chlamydia, or HIV (Wawer et al., 1999). Reductions in STI prevalence were observed in Masaka, Uganda, where the prevalence of active syphilis (RR = 0.52; 95 percent CI 0.27–0.98) and gonorrhoea (RR = 0.25; 95 percent CI 0.10–0.64) was lower in the syndromic management and information, education, and communication (IEC) arm (but not in the IEC-alone arm) compared with the control arm. However, there was no concomitant reduction in chlamydia prevalence and HIV incidence (Kamali et al., 2003). A trial of syndromic STI management and a peer-led targeted behavior change and condom promotion intervention in Manicaland, rural Zimbabwe, showed no impact on HIV incidence and no difference in reported STI syndromes (Gregson et al., 2007). A community RCT of adolescent sexual health interventions in Tanzania showed no impact on biological outcomes (Ross et al., 2007).

STI control programs can decrease HIV incidence under certain programmatic settings and epidemic circumstances. Many negative trials following the promising original Mwanza study have suggested that the intervention in isolation is not robust in diminishing HIV incidence. Nevertheless, the role of STI control remains relevant for multicomponent interventions and should be studied further (Grosskurth et al., 2000; Tanton et al., 2010).

Evidence of What Works from National Trends

While the results of RCTs are disappointing or inconclusive, observations of population trends in HIV incidence and associated risk behaviors tell a different story, revealing that substantial reductions in risk behaviors have led to detectable reductions in HIV prevalence. Sentinel surveillance data, along with cohort studies in Uganda, provided the first African example of such national successes (Kilian et al., 1999; Stoneburner and Low-Beer, 2004). Subsequently, similar reductions were observed in Zimbabwe (Gregson et al., 2006) and Kenya (Hallett et al., 2006). More recently, a review of trends in prevalence among 15- to 24-year-olds either attending antenatal clinics or participating in household-based surveys used as a marker of recent incidence rates[2] found reductions in Botswana, Côte d'Ivoire, Ethiopia, Kenya, Malawi, Namibia, Zimbabwe, Zambia, South Africa, and Tanzania (International Group on Analysis of Trends in HIV Prevalence and Behaviours in Young People in Countries Most Affected by HIV, 2010). These findings demonstrate that HIV/AIDS prevention is possible. In other countries, there may have been reductions in incidence that cannot be distinguished from the expected saturation and stabilization in prevalence.

Unfortunately, identifying the sufficient or necessary conditions for national programs to attain such measurable success has not been possible. What distinguishes countries with and without declines in incidence is not certain. Retrospective analysis suggests that major shifts in the attitudes of populations are required, with information coming from trusted sources in a social and cultural environment rather than specific programmed activity. An analysis linking the intensity of intervention activities and declines in prevalence is not possible since the effort or expenditure preceding the changes has not been documented. If we take a more recent measure of expenditure to be representative of past expenditure, we might expect a relationship. Even when controlling for initial prevalence, however, there appears to be no relationship between expenditure and the scale of reductions in prevalence. Figure 2-1 shows that there is no discernible association between HIV/AIDS prevention spending per person and the degree of improvement in HIV prevalence among young people.

Is There Scope for Greater Effort?

Despite the substantial observed reductions in risk achieved in African countries with generalized epidemics, the levels of HIV incidence in Africa remain high compared with those in other regions. In Zimbabwe, for example, it has been estimated that incidence dropped by 40 percent in urban residents between 1999 and 2004—from around 5 percent per year to 3 percent per year (Hallett et al., 2009). In no African country has prevalence in 15- to 24-year-olds fallen

---

[2] Data on prevalence in 15- to 24-year-olds are used as a proxy for incidence.

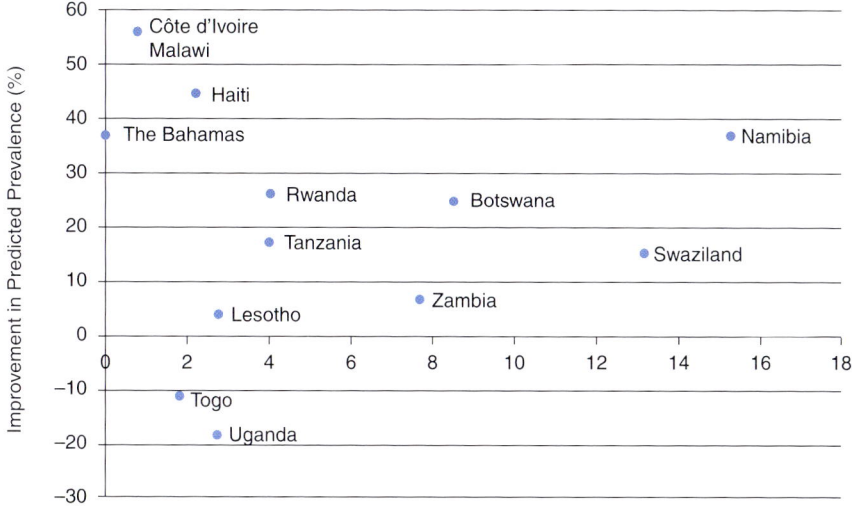

FIGURE 2-1 No obvious association is discernable between aggregate expenditure on prevention of HIV and degree of prevalence decline in countries where decline has been observed.
SOURCE: Committee's calculations using prevalence data from International Group on Analysis of Trends in HIV Prevalence and Behaviours in Young People in Countries Most Affected by HIV (2010) and expenditure data from UNAIDS epidemic update (UNAIDS, 2008).

below 1 percent. Thus, even where prevention effects reduce the long-term burden of HIV/AIDS, the rate of new infections is still likely to outstrip even modestly ambitious rates of treatment uptake. Prospects for reducing incidence over the long term are more promising, however.

Figure 2-2 shows the results of a model constructed by the committee that assumes optimistically that the uptake rate of 30 percent of unmet need for treatment attained in 2007–2009 is sustained at WHO's new definition of need,[3] but with no additional prevention success, while donor support for treatment increases. For 2020, this model projects about 20 million people on treatment (Panel a) and treatment costs alone of about $15 billion (Panel c), with both measures of burden continuing to rise thereafter until reaching 50 million on treatment and $40 billion per year for treatment by 2050. In the absence of improved prevention, the number of new infections rises from 2 million per year currently to

---

[3] In 2010, WHO revised its AIDS treatment guidelines to recommend treatment initiation when the CD4 count drops below 350, greatly expanding its estimate of the number of people in need of treatment.

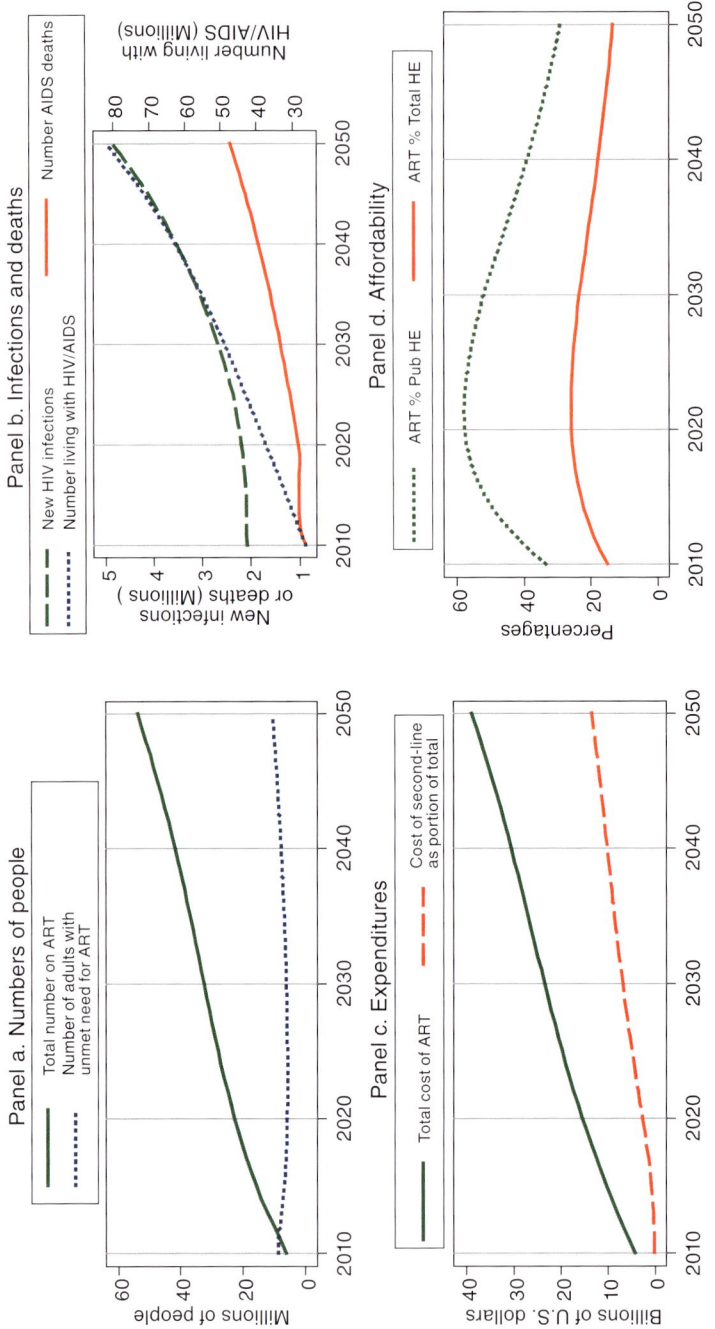

FIGURE 2-2 Assuming increased donor support for treatment without additional prevention, the committee projects for 2020 about 20 million people on treatment and treatment costs alone of about $15 billion.

SOURCE: Committee projections using data from UNAIDS (2008).

NOTE: Pub HE stands for public health expenditure and Total HE stands for total health expenditure.

2.3 million per year in 2020 and almost 5 million per year in 2050 (Panel b, left axis). While treatment expansion succeeds in holding AIDS mortality down to its current level of about 1 million per year through 2020, mortality then begins to rise as a result of the combined effects of accumulating new infections and the eventual deaths of those begun on treatment through 2020, so that annual deaths double to more than 2 million in 2050. With the annual number of new cases being twice as large as the number of deaths through 2020 and a growing multiple of deaths thereafter, the total number of people living with HIV/AIDS grows to 40 million in 2020 and then doubles to 80 million by 2050 (Panel b, right axis). Panel d of Figure 2-2 provides another perspective on the same total cost of HIV/AIDS treatment shown in Panel c, charting its evolution as a percentage of two measures of total African resource availability—total public health expenditure and total public and private health expenditure. Using World Bank estimates of future African economic growth rates and assuming that these expenditures grow at the same rate as the overall economies, the model predicts that after reaching peaks of about 60 percent of public and 25 percent of total health spending in 2020, these measures of burden will begin to improve as economic growth begins to outstrip the growth in treatment cost.

Figure 2-3 uses the same model as Figure 2-2 with the new WHO definition of need for treatment and 30 percent uptake of unmet need, but it assumes that male circumcision is successfully expanded to cover 90 percent of African men by 2025. Under these assumptions, increased donor support for treatment leads to 22 million on treatment at an annual cost of about $15 billion in 2020, about the same burden as in Figure 2-2 without the success of male circumcision, but the longer-term prospect is improved. As can be seen in Panel b of Figure 2-3, the impact of enhanced prevention is to slowly reduce the annual number of new infections until in 2030, it is less than the number of deaths from AIDS, and the number of people living with HIV/AIDS begins to decline.[4] As a result of the momentum of the 27 million people surviving on treatment in 2030, the cost of HIV/AIDS treatment only levels off in absolute terms, but it does begin to decline after 2030 relative to projected African governments' health expenditures.

Figure 2-4 shows the impact of adding other extremely effective prevention interventions to the successful male circumcision modeled in Figure 2-3. Assuming that by 2025 these other interventions reduce the HIV incidence rate to only 30 percent of what it would otherwise have been has little effect on the projected burden of the epidemic in 2020, but it has a dramatic effect by 2050. Because the number of people living with HIV/AIDS begins to decline in 2020, the number of people on treatment begins to decline in 2028, and by 2050, the annual cost of HIV/AIDS treatment has declined from its peak to about one-third less, with an annual cost of around $15 billion per year by 2050 compared with

---

[4] This milestone has been dubbed the "AIDS Transition" (Over, 2010) and could be considered an important intermediate objective on the way to universal treatment coverage.

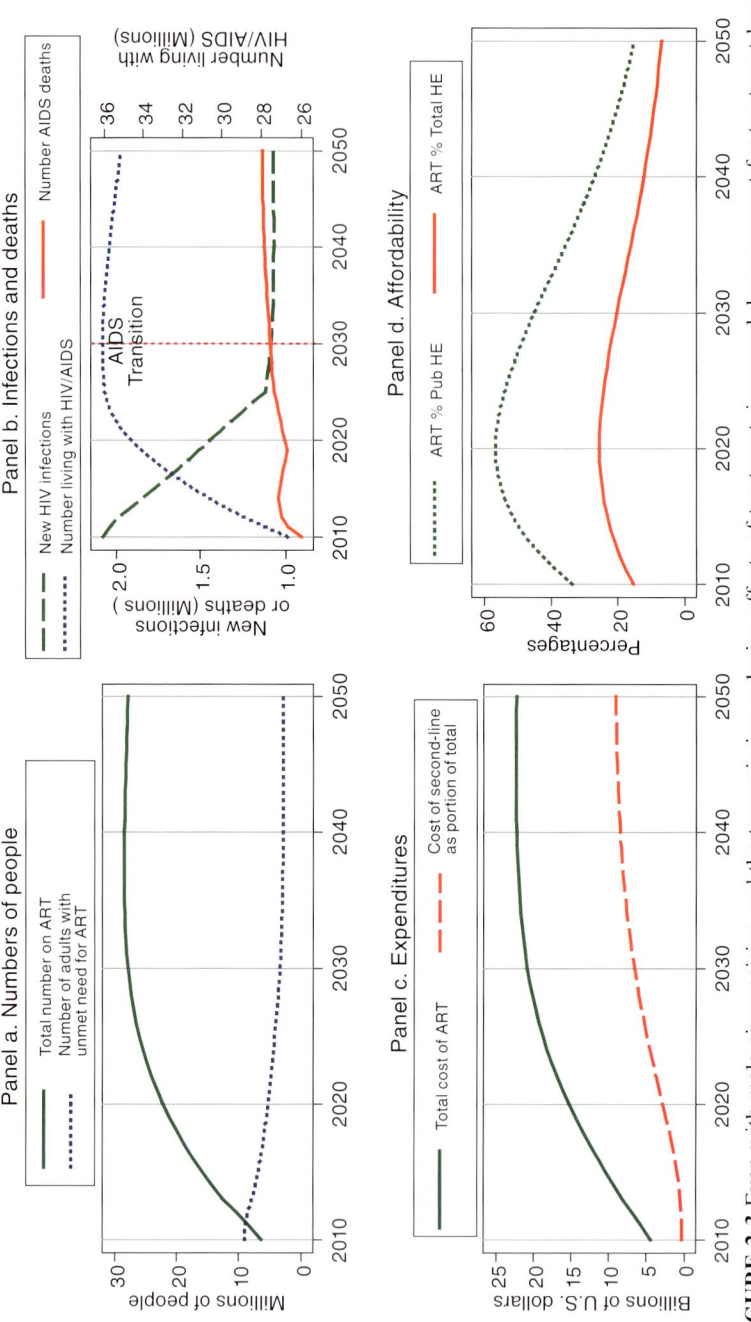

FIGURE 2-3 Even with male circumcision and the transmission-reducing effects of treatment, increased donor support for treatment leads to 22 million on treatment at an annual cost of about $15 billion in 2020, but the numbers living with HIV/AIDS begin to decline in 2030.

SOURCE: Committee calculations using data from UNAIDS (2008).

NOTE: Pub HE stands for public health expenditure and Total HE stands for total health expenditure.

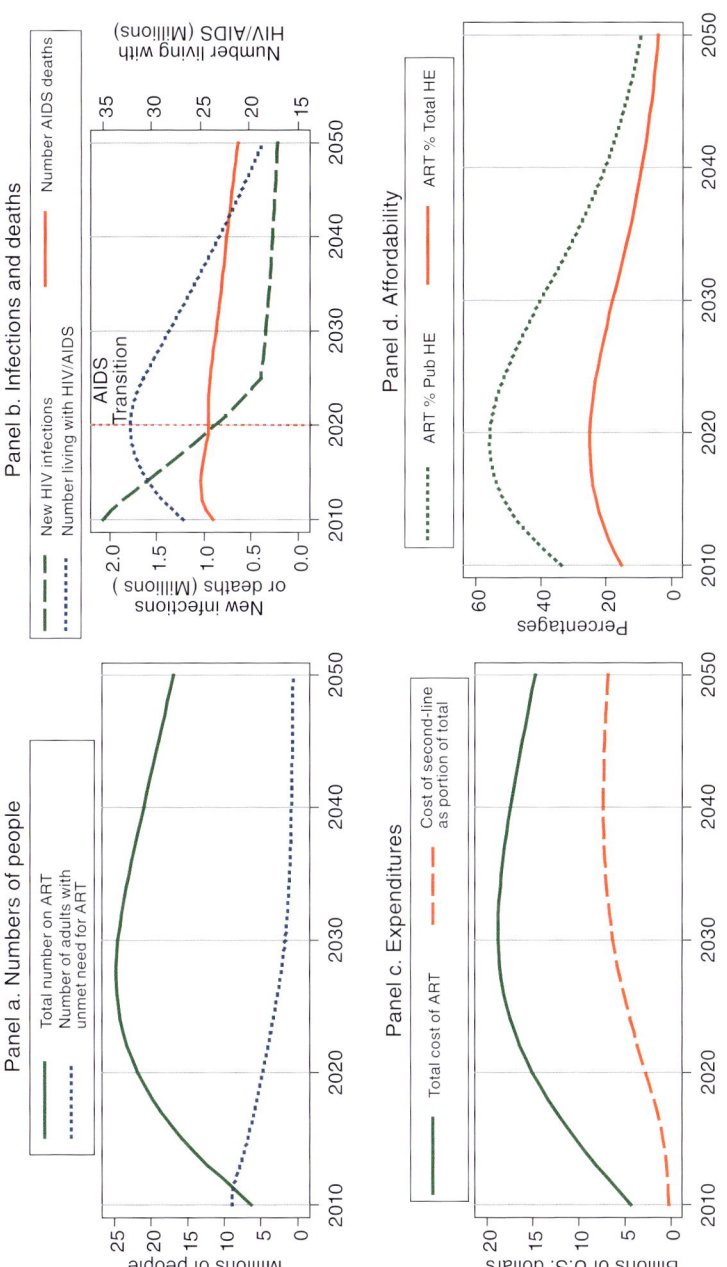

FIGURE 2-4 Given increased donor support and major prevention efforts, the committee projects reduced treatment need and reduced costs in 2050.

SOURCE: Committee calculations using data from UNAIDS (2008).

NOTE: Pub HE stands for public health expenditure and Total HE stands for total health expenditure.

about $23 billion per year at its peak around 2028. Furthermore, after peaking at almost 60 percent of health spending in 2020, the total cost of ART declines to about 10 percent of government health spending in 2050.

Given current trends to slow the recruitment of new patients to treatment and to proceed cautiously in recruiting patients before they have symptoms, treatment costs may be substantially reduced by 2020. Figure 2-5 presents one of the most plausible, if less optimistic, scenarios for 2020. In response to its statement of task, the committee designates this the "best" projection of the HIV/AIDS incidence and burden in Africa. It assumes that recent rates of uptake of about 10 percent of those with unmet need are sustained each year. This 10 percent uptake rate is less than the 30 percent rate achieved between 2007 and 2009, but roughly consonant with PEPFAR's current goal of 4 million on treatment by 2014. This scenario also assumes that the median threshold CD4 count for treatment initiation remains as it is today, at about 130, and that prevention efforts remain modest, with circumcision reaching only 10 percent of African men by 2025. With this parsimonious approach to treatment and in the absence of improved prevention, the total number of patients on treatment in 2020 reaches 7 million in Africa, and annual expenditures for treatment total approximately $7 billion. The number of people living with HIV/AIDS continues to rise in the coming decades, reaching 70 million by 2050, when annual costs for HIV/AIDS treatment are more than $12 billion per year. The only positive note is that total costs are likely to decline as a proportion of total government health spending, on the assumption that African economies grow at the 4 to 5 percent rates that are projected for the next several years (The World Bank, 2010).

Thus, by 2050, there is little difference in annual treatment costs between the Figure 2-5 scenario of parsimonious treatment without prevention and the scenario of Figure 2-4 with increased donor support and strong HIV/AIDS prevention. The difference between the two is in the intervening cost profile (continuously falling as a percentage of government health spending in Figure 2-5 versus a sharp rise followed by a fall to the equivalent level in Figure 2-4), and in the numbers of and trend in deaths (in 2050, 3 million and rising in Figure 2-5 versus 700,000 and falling in Figure 2-4). Thus, donors resolve to bear a larger proportion of treatment costs, if accompanied by a sufficiently effective prevention effort, can improve the situation in Africa by 2050 relative to a more parsimonious strategy.

Under several plausible scenarios, then, while total HIV/AIDS treatment costs will continue to rise (because a larger share of people will be on more expensive second-line medications), they will eventually decline as a proportion of the health budgets of African countries. This decline will occur immediately if scale-up is parsimonious. Even with more generous scale-up, however, continued growth of the African economies at rates similar to those seen in the last decade, together with improved HIV/AIDS prevention, can produce a decline in HIV/AIDS treatment costs as a percentage of domestic health care spending after 2020

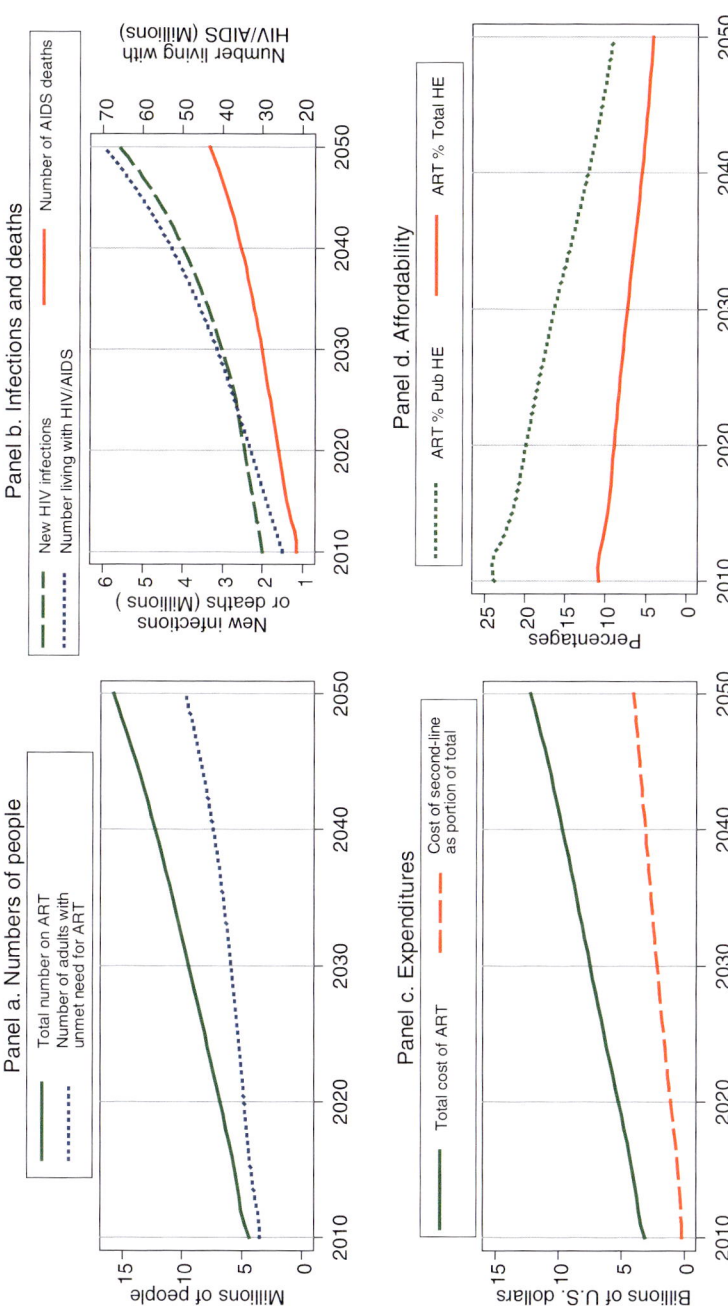

FIGURE 2-5 A plausible "best" projection for the future, assuming a parsimonious approach to treatment scale-up and no improvement in prevention efficacy, showing 7 million on treatment at an annual cost of $7 billion in 2020.

SOURCE: Committee projections using data from UNAIDS (2008).

NOTE: Pub HE stands for public health expenditure and Total HE stands for total health expenditure.

or 2025. Should this decline occur, African governments will be able to move toward greater ownership of their countries' HIV/AIDS prevention, treatment, and care objectives in the foreseeable future.

Beyond the impact of behavior changes already observed, there might be benefits of expanding prevention efforts. Using interventions with observed efficacy in improving either HIV incidence or intermediate outcomes, we can calculate the predicted impact of prevention interventions, including high coverage of counseling and testing and adult male circumcision. Again the impact is substantial, but falls short of what might be described as controlling the spread of HIV/AIDS. Further reductions are possible, however, if infectiousness is reduced by expanding treatment and if we assume that this expansion leads to no increase in risk behavior (see the next section). The efficacy of a tenofovir vaginal microbicide and developments in vaccines (including the identification of broadly neutralizing antibodies) hold promise for providing additional prevention tools that would further reduce HIV incidence. In addition, structural interventions may be able to play a role. The success of individually oriented interventions in reducing risk behavior is substantially improved when prevention addresses the broader structural factors that shape or constrain individual behavior, such as poverty and wealth, gender, age, policy, and power (Gupta et al., 2008). In combination, these interventions may be able to dramatically reduce HIV incidence.

POTENTIAL FOR REDUCING TREATMENT NEED

If HIV incidence can be dramatically reduced so that more individuals are receiving treatment than are becoming newly infected, the need to initiate treatment will eventually start to decline. Given that treatment is a form of prevention, the earlier during the course of their infection individuals are initiated on treatment, the sooner this reduction in need for treatment will be realized.

It has been argued that a dramatic expansion of testing and immediate initiation of treatment in a "test and treat" strategy could reduce incidence to less than 0.1 percent per year (Burns et al., 2010; Dieffenbach and Fauci, 2009; Granich et al., 2009). The strategy modeled involved annual testing and assumed a 50 percent reduction in risk behavior to generate this optimistic scenario. The observed reduction in transmission in discordant couples in the context of an RCT—93 percent—will likely be less in normal treatment programs, where adherence may be lower and treatment failure more common. Nonetheless, observational studies suggest that the viral load associated with treatment generates the reduced transmissibility expected from studies of transmission as a function of viral load (Quinn et al., 2000; Semaye Fideli et al., 2001). Subsequent modeling work incorporating heterogeneities in risk behavior and greater transmissibility associated with primary viraemia suggests that reductions in incidence may be less than those in an initial model but would still be important.

Unfortunately, the effort required to ensure such regular testing and immediate treatment would be great and beyond anything that has been achieved even in developed countries. Furthermore, there is a concern that increases in risk behavior seen in some developed countries among those receiving treatment and others in their communities (Fisher et al., 2004) could also occur in the heterosexual populations of Africa. To counter this concern, data from South Africa suggest dramatic reductions in risk behavior associated with receiving ART (Venkatesh et al., 2010). Unfortunately, excluding biases in reporting is difficult in such clinical settings. In addition, the behavior of those with a diagnosed HIV infection may be less relevant than the behavior of susceptible individuals and those whose infection is undiagnosed who may continue to spread the virus.

Despite these concerns, there may be a role for treatment as prevention, especially if future regimens can be made to be more easily administered and monitored, with fewer toxicities and simpler dosing. This is an aspiration of UNAIDS laid out in Treatment 2.0 (UNAIDS, 2010). Exploring the relationship among viral load and transmissibility, CD4 count, and period from infection to different CD4 counts, we can calculate the expected proportion of new HIV infections generated by infectious individuals before they start treatment. The earlier treatment begins, the greater the proportion of these infections we would expect to be averted. With approximately a third of new infections being associated with contact with those with a CD4 count below 200, we can expect good treatment coverage to impact the spread of HIV/AIDS, adding to the effect of other prevention interventions.

It should be noted that the optimism surrounding the prevention impact of treatment should be tempered by the distinct lack of population-level empirical evidence. One recent study linked the current diagnosis of HIV infections (presumably a delayed measure of incidence) to the current coverage of treatment (Montaner et al., 2010), but the interpretation of these data is controversial.

It should also be noted that, if earlier treatment is expanded, this obviously means that many more people will need to be on treatment in the short term. The decline in numbers requiring treatment will be gradual, with a pattern reflecting the distribution of periods from infection to treatment need. Using the median of approximately 9 years from HIV acquisition to a CD4 count of 200, with variation depending on age, prior health condition, and other factors (Aalen et al., 1997; Van Der Paal et al., 2007), the lag will be on the order of a decade. Thus any reduction in incidence achieved in 2010 will be only partially realized by 2020, and the benefits of reduced incidence need to be considered over a period of decades.

KEY POLICY CHOICES AND ASSOCIATED TRADE-OFFS

The burden of HIV/AIDS is extremely sensitive to alternative policies. Competing activities can consume available resources; the effects of these various activities need to be compared and the trade-offs considered to guide decisions about optimum strategies.

Early Versus Late Treatment Initiation

Treatment initiation at a higher CD4 count leads to a better prognosis for those receiving treatment, and as noted above, the WHO guidelines have shifted to recommend earlier treatment. This means that each person treated receives the treatment for a longer period, potentially reducing the treatment available to others—presumably the thinking behind many countries not implementing the WHO guidelines.

Over the short term, allocating a fixed number of treatment slots to sicker patients should save more lives since those being treated would otherwise be near death. Over the longer term, the reduced treatment failure seen with early treatment could reduce the numbers of deaths and increase years of life saved. The optimum time for treatment initiation will therefore depend on the horizon over which benefits are calculated and the discounting that is used to weigh future costs and benefits against current costs and benefits.

In addition to changing the criteria for initiation, the new WHO treatment guidelines recommend the more expensive, less toxic tenofovir. The trade-off between this clinically preferred, more expensive regimen and a poorer, cheaper regimen is one of greater benefit for fewer treated patients.

Coverage with Second-Line Versus First-Line Regimens

Those failing first-line treatment require second-line regimens if they are to continue on treatment. Given that these second-line regimens are more expensive than first-line regimens, more people can be put on the latter for the same cost. Thus, the improved survival of treated patients if a second-line regimen is available should be weighed against the number of people that could benefit from first-line regimens.

Quality Versus Quantity of Programs:
Follow-Up, Adherence, and Virological Tests

Similar trade-offs must be considered with respect to expensive programs that invest in following up to ensure that patients are maintained within the program, in promoting and ensuring adherence of patients, and in using laboratory tests to identify treatment failure. Virological measures allow treatment failure to be identified sooner than is possible through observation of symptoms, enabling second-line regimens to replace failing first-line regimens. In addition to improving survival, this approach has the benefit of preventing a failing regimen from leading to greater drug resistance. An alternative to second-line regimens is to withdraw treatment. This approach would likely reduce survival, but would concomitantly reduce the expense of wasted treatment and the selective pressures on the virus.

Investment in Prevention Versus Treatment

Whether to invest in prevention or treatment has been a recurrent theme in debates about priorities in controlling HIV/AIDS. This trade-off was explicit in the earmarking of funds in the original President's Emergency Plan for AIDS Relief (PEPFAR) authorization. To explore a trade-off between the benefits of treatment and prevention assumes that they achieve different results. As discussed in the preceding section, however, there is consensus that the two can have a synergistic effect. ART can reduce HIV transmission both directly (by reducing viraemia and thereby HIV transmissibility) and indirectly (by reducing risk behavior among those diagnosed, counseled, and treated and by diffusing attitudes and norms among the population that facilitate a general acceptance of the problem of HIV/AIDS and changes in risk behavior). However, resources and effort are required to realize the prevention benefits of treatment and to avoid unintended consequences of treatment, such as increased risk behavior. Resources are required to build on the hope created by treatment to change behavioral norms among patients and in the larger community. A further reason to link these programs is that advocates of faster treatment uptake can use evidence of prevention success to lobby for more treatment resources.

These potential complementarities between prevention and treatment suggest the need for a strategy that builds on both rather than trading them off. However, separation of the resources available and responsibility for the two means they are likely to be traded off and to compete for resources.

RECOMMENDATIONS

Given the enormous momentum of the HIV/AIDS epidemic, even a large increase in prevention effort and effectiveness over the next few years can have little impact on the mortality or financial burden of HIV/AIDS before 2020. By changing the future course of the epidemic, however, greatly improved HIV/AIDS prevention can dramatically reduce the financial burden of donor and recipient governments beyond 2020. Donors and governments that experience success in reducing new infections to the extent that the total number living with HIV/AIDS begins to fall can reasonably expect treatment expenditures to decline beyond 2020 and therefore can afford to invest some of those future savings in a greater rate of patient enrollment today.

Recommendation 2-1[5]: *Measure incidence.* African countries, with the support of donors, should develop and implement cost-effective methods for accurately measuring the level of and change in HIV/AIDS incidence to enable better planning and evaluation of HIV/AIDS prevention programs.[6]

Recommendation 2-2: *Analyze trade-offs.* The U.S. government should support countries in developing projections of the future burden of their HIV/AIDS epidemics and in assessing the implications of alternative national HIV/AIDS policies for human welfare, capacity, and resources so policy makers can make informed decisions on HIV/AIDS-related trade-offs.

REFERENCES

Aalen, O. O., V. T. Farewell, D. De Angelis, N. E. Day, and O. N. Gill. 1997. A Markov model for HIV disease progression including the effect of HIV diagnosis and treatment: Application to AIDS prediction in England and Wales. *Statistics in Medicine* 16(19):2191-2210.

Auvert, B., D. Taljaard, E. Lagarde, J. Sobngwi-Tambekou, R. Sitta, and A. Puren. 2005. Randomized, controlled intervention trial of male circumcision for reduction of HIV infection risk: The ANRS 1265 trial. *PLoS Medicine* 2(11):e298.

Bailey, R. C., S. Moses, C. B. Parker, K. Agot, I. Maclean, J. N. Krieger, C. F. Williams, R. T. Campbell, and J. O. Ndinya-Achola. 2007. Male circumcision for HIV prevention in young men in Kisumu, Kenya: A randomised controlled trial. *The Lancet* 369(9562):643-656.

Burns, D. N., C. W. Dieffenbach, and S. H. Vermund. 2010. Rethinking prevention of HIV type 1 infection. *Clinical Infectious Diseases* 51(6):725-731.

Busch, M., C. Pilcher, T. Mastro, J. Kaldor, G. Vercauteren, W. Rodriguez, C. Rousseau, T. Rehle, A. Welte, M. Averill, and J. Calleja. 2010. Beyond detuning: 10 years of progress and new challenges in the development and application of assays for HIV incidence estimation. *AIDS* 24(18):2763-2771.

Connor, E. M., R. S. Sperling, R. Gelber, P. Kiselev, G. Scott, M. J. O'Sullivan, R. Vandyke, M. Bey, W. Shearer, R. L. Jacobson, E. Jimenez, E. O'Neill, B. Bazin, J. F. Delfraissy, M. Culnane, R. Coombs, M. Elkins, J. Moye, P. Stratton, and J. Balsley. 1994. Reduction of maternal-infant transmission of human immunodeficiency virus type 1 with zidovudine treatment. *The New England Journal of Medicine* 331(18):1173-1180.

Dieffenbach, C. W., and A. S. Fauci. 2009. Universal voluntary testing and treatment for prevention of HIV transmission. *Journal of the American Medical Association* 301(22):2380-2382.

Fiamma, A., P. Lissouba, O. E. Amy, B. Singh, O. Laeyendecker, T. C. Quinn, D. Taljaard, and B. Auvert. 2010. Can HIV incidence testing be used for evaluating HIV intervention programs? A reanalysis of the Orange Farm male circumcision trial (ANRS-1265). *BMC Infectious Diseases* 10:137.

---

[5] The committee's recommendations are numbered according to the chapters of the report in which they appear. Thus, for example, recommendation 2-1 is the first recommendation in Chapter 2.

[6] As described in Chapter 2, laboratory-based assays for the calculation of incidence estimates are in development and are urgently needed to provide important epidemiological data on trends of the epidemic and the effectiveness of interventions so that limited resources can be directed most efficiently to limit the epidemic's further spread.

Fisher, J. D., D. H. Cornman, C. Y. Osborn, K. R. Amico, W. A. Fisher, and G. A. Friedland. 2004. Clinician-initiated HIV risk reduction intervention for HIV-positive persons: Formative research, acceptability, and fidelity of the Options Project. *Journal of Acquired Immune Deficiency Syndromes (1999)* 37(Suppl. 2):S78-S87.

Granich, R. M., C. F. Gilks, C. Dye, K. M. De Cock, and B. G. Williams. 2009. Universal voluntary HIV testing with immediate antiretroviral therapy as a strategy for elimination of HIV transmission: A mathematical model. *The Lancet* 373(9657):48-57.

Gray, R. H., G. Kigozi, D. Serwadda, F. Makumbi, S. Watya, F. Nalugoda, N. Kiwanuka, L. H. Moulton, M. A. Chaudhary, M. Z. Chen, N. K. Sewankambo, F. Wabwire-Mangen, M. C. Bacon, C. F. Williams, P. Opendi, S. J. Reynolds, O. Laeyendecker, T. C. Quinn, and M. J. Wawer. 2007. Male circumcision for HIV prevention in men in Rakai, Uganda: A randomised trial. *The Lancet* 369(9562):657-666.

Gregson, S., S. Adamson, S. Papaya, J. Mundondo, C. A. Nyamukapa, P. R. Mason, G. P. Garnett, S. K. Chandiwana, G. Foster, and R. M. Anderson. 2007. Impact and process evaluation of integrated community and clinic-based HIV-1 control: A cluster-randomised trial in eastern Zimbabwe. *PLoS Medicine* 4(3):e102.

Gregson, S., G. P. Garnett, C. A. Nyamukapa, T. B. Hallett, J. J. Lewis, P. R. Mason, S. K. Chandiwana, and R. M. Anderson. 2006. HIV decline associated with behavior change in eastern Zimbabwe. *Science* 311(5761):664-666.

Grosskurth, H., F. Mosha, J. Todd, E. Mwijarubi, A. Klokke, K. Senkoro, P. Mayaud, J. Changalucha, A. Nicoll, G. ka-Gina, J. Newell, K. Mugeye, D. Mabey, and R. Hayes. 1995. Impact of improved treatment of sexually transmitted diseases on HIV infection in rural Tanzania: Randomised controlled trial. *The Lancet* 346(8974):530-536.

Grosskurth, H., E. Mwijarubi, J. Todd, M. Rwakatare, K. Orroth, P. Mayaud, B. Cleophas, A. Buvé, R. Mkanje, L. Ndeki, A. Gavyole, R. Hayes, and D. Mabey. 2000. Operational performance of an STD control programme in Mwanza Region, Tanzania. *Sexually Transmitted Infections* 76(6):426-436.

Gupta, G. R., J. O. Parkhurst, J. A. Ogden, P. Aggleton, and A. Mahal. 2008. Structural approaches to HIV prevention. *The Lancet* 372(9640):764-775.

Hallett, T. B., J. Aberle-Grasse, G. Bello, L. M. Boulos, M. P. Cayemittes, B. Cheluget, J. Chipeta, R. Dorrington, S. Dube, A. K. Ekra, J. M. Garcia-Calleja, G. P. Garnett, S. Greby, S. Gregson, J. T. Grove, S. Hader, J. Hanson, W. Hladik, S. Ismail, S. Kassim, W. Kirungi, L. Kouassi, A. Mahomva, L. Marum, C. Maurice, M. Nolan, T. Rehle, J. Stover, and N. Walker. 2006. Declines in HIV prevalence can be associated with changing sexual behaviour in Uganda, urban Kenya, Zimbabwe, and urban Haiti. *Sexually Transmitted Infections* 82(Suppl. 1):i1-i8.

Hallett, T. B., S. Gregson, E. Gonese, O. Mugurungi, and G. P. Garnett. 2009. Assessing evidence for behaviour change affecting the course of HIV epidemics: A new mathematical modelling approach and application to data from Zimbabwe. *Epidemics* 1:108-117.

International Group on Analysis of Trends in HIV Prevalence and Behaviours in Young People in Countries Most Affected by HIV. 2010. Trends in HIV prevalence and sexual behaviour among young people aged 15-24 years in countries most affected by HIV. *Journal of Sexually Transmitted Infections* 86(Suppl 2):ii72-ii83.

Kamali, A., M. Quigley, J. Nakiyingi, J. Kinsman, J. Kengeya-Kayondo, R. Gopal, A. Ojwiya, P. Hughes, L. M. Carpenter, and J. Whitworth. 2003. Syndromic management of sexually-transmitted infections and behaviour change interventions on transmission of HIV-1 in rural Uganda: A community randomised trial. *The Lancet* 361(9358):645-652.

Karim, Q. A., S. S. Karim, J. A. Frohlich, A. C. Grobler, C. Baxter, L. E. Mansoor, A. B. Kharsany, S. Sibeko, K. P. Mlisana, Z. Omar, T. N. Gengiah, S. Maarschalk, N. Arulappan, M. Mlotshwa, L. Morris, and D. Taylor. 2010. Effectiveness and safety of tenofovir gel, an antiretroviral microbicide, for the prevention of HIV infection in women. *Science* 329(5996)1168-1174.

Kilian, A. H., S. Gregson, B. Ndyanabangi, K. Walusaga, W. Kipp, G. Sahlmuller, G. P. Garnett, G. Asiimwe-Okiror, G. Kabagambe, P. Weis, and F. von Sonnenburg. 1999. Reductions in risk behaviour provide the most consistent explanation for declining HIV-1 prevalence in Uganda. *AIDS* 13(3):391-398.

Mastro, T. D., A. A. Kim, T. Hallett, T. Rehle, A. Welte, O. Laeyendecker, T. Oluoch, and J. M. Garcia-Calleja. 2010. Estimating HIV incidence in populations using tests for recent infection: Issues, challenges and the way forward. *Journal of HIV/AIDS Surveillance & Epidemiology* 2(1).

Montaner, J. S., V. D. Lima, R. Barrios, B. Yip, E. Wood, T. Kerr, K. Shannon, P. R. Harrigan, R. S. Hogg, P. Daly, and P. Kendall. 2010. Association of highly active antiretroviral therapy coverage, population viral load, and yearly new HIV diagnoses in British Columbia, Canada: A population-based study. *The Lancet* 376(9740):532-539.

Over, M. 2010. *The global AIDS transition: A feasible objective for AIDS policy.* Washington, DC: Center for Global Development.

Padian, N. S., S. I. McCoy, J. E. Balkus, and J. N. Wasserheit. 2010. Weighing the gold in the gold standard: Challenges in HIV prevention research. *AIDS* 24(5):621-635.

Quinn, T. C., M. J. Wawer, N. Sewankambo, D. Serwadda, C. Li, F. Wabwire-Mangen, M. O. Meehan, T. Lutalo, and R. H. Gray. 2000. Viral load and heterosexual transmission of human immunodeficiency virus type 1. Rakai Project Study Group. *The New England Journal of Medicine* 342(13):921-929.

Rerks-Ngarm, S., P. Pitisuttithum, S. Nitayaphan, J. Kaewkungwal, J. Chiu, R. Paris, N. Premsri, C. Namwat, M. de Souza, E. Adams, M. Benenson, S. Gurunathan, J. Tartaglia, J. G. McNeil, D. P. Francis, D. Stablein, D. L. Birx, S. Chunsuttiwat, C. Khamboonruang, P. Thongcharoen, M. L. Robb, N. L. Michael, P. Kunasol, and J. H. Kim. 2009. Vaccination with ALVAC and AIDSVAX to prevent HIV-1 infection in Thailand. *The New England Journal of Medicine* 361(23):2209-2220.

Ross, D. A., J. Changalucha, A. I. Obasi, J. Todd, M. L. Plummer, B. Cleophas-Mazige, A. Anemona, D. Everett, H. A. Weiss, D. C. Mabey, H. Grosskurth, and R. J. Hayes. 2007. Biological and behavioural impact of an adolescent sexual health intervention in Tanzania: A community-randomized trial. *AIDS* 21(14):1943-1955.

Semaye Fideli, U., S. A. Allen, R. Musonda, S. Trask, B. H. Hahn, H. Weiss, J. Mulenga, F. Kasolo, S. H. Vermund, and G. M. Aldrovand. 2001. Virologic and immunologic determinants of heterosexual transmission of human immunodeficiency virus type 1 in Africa. *AIDS Research and Human Retroviruses* 17(10):901-910.

Stoneburner, R. L., and D. Low-Beer. 2004. Population-level HIV declines and behavioral risk avoidance in Uganda. *Science* 304(5671):714-718.

Susser, M. 1996. Some principles in study design for preventing HIV transmission: Rigor or reality. *American Journal of Public Health* 86(12):1713-1716.

Tanton, C., H. A. Weiss, J. Rusizoka, J. LeGoff, J. Changalucha, K. Baisley, K. Mugeye, D. Everett, L. Belec, T. C. Clayton, D. A. Ross, R. J. Hayes, and D. Watson-Jones. 2010. Long-term impact of acyclovir suppressive therapy on genital and plasma HIV RNA in Tanzanian women: A randomized controlled trial. *The Journal of Infectious Diseases* 201(9):1285-1297.

UNAIDS (The Joint United Nations Programme on HIV/AIDS). 2008. *Report on the global AIDS epidemic.* Geneva: UNAIDS.

———. 2010. *Fact sheet: Treatment 2.0.* Geneva: UNAIDS.

Van Der Paal, L., L. A. Shafer, J. Todd, B. N. Mayanja, J. A. Whitworth, and H. Grosskurth. 2007. HIV-1 disease progression and mortality before the introduction of highly active antiretroviral therapy in rural Uganda. *AIDS* 21(Suppl. 6):S21-S29.

Venkatesh, K. K., G. de Bruyn, M. N. Lurie, L. Mohapi, P. Pronyk, M. Moshabela, E. Marinda, G. E. Gray, E. W. Triche, and N. A. Martinson. 2010. Decreased sexual risk behavior in the era of HAART among HIV-infected urban and rural South Africans attending primary care clinics. *Journal of Acquired Immune Deficiency Syndromes* 24.

Wawer, M. J., N. K. Sewankambo, D. Serwadda, T. C. Quinn, L. A. Paxton, N. Kiwanuka, F. Wabwire-Mangen, C. Li, T. Lutalo, F. Nalugoda, C. A. Gaydos, L. H. Moulton, M. O. Meehan, S. Ahmed, and R. H. Gray. 1999. Control of sexually transmitted diseases for AIDS prevention in Uganda: A randomised community trial. Rakai Project Study Group. *The Lancet* 353(9152):525-535.

Welte, A., T. A. McWalter, O. Laeyendecker, and T. B. Hallett. 2010. Using tests for recent infection to estimate incidence: Problems and prospects for HIV. *Eurosurveillance* 15(24).

The World Bank. 2010. *Global economic prospects: Fiscal headwinds and recovery.* Washington, DC: The World Bank.

3

The Burden of HIV/AIDS:
Implications for U.S. Interests

Key Findings

- The expected growth in the burden of HIV/AIDS in the coming decade portends significant challenges for the United States in sustaining and expanding commitments to combating HIV/AIDS in Africa.
- The combination of competing health and development demands, the rising cost burden of HIV/AIDS treatment, and continued resource constraints will force difficult choices and trade-offs for U.S. policy makers, made more politically sensitive by heightened expectations around U.S. commitments to HIV/AIDS prevention, treatment, and care services in Africa.
- The epidemic in Africa is a crisis that requires both an emergency response and the forethought, planning, and sustained commitment of a long-term development intervention. Accordingly, the international community must focus now on preventive measures and human and institutional capacity building.
- Strategies for addressing the impacts of the epidemic on U.S. interests include moving toward shared responsibility with African partner states, leveraging multilateral assets, and striving for integration and efficiency.

The HIV/AIDS epidemic, first identified in 1981, remains among the greatest threats to global health, with an epicenter in the acutely affected countries of east and southern Africa (Independent Task Force Report No. 56, 2006; UNAIDS and WHO, 2009). Life-saving antiretroviral therapy (ART) was, until 2000, not accessible to those most in need because they were poor and lived in developing countries. With the turn of the 21st century, global attitudes on this morally intolerable situation began to shift, and the International AIDS Conference in Durban in July 2000 marked a turning point with a powerful call to the international community to take responsibility for mounting an urgent response.

The United States responded and, with the launch of the U.S. President's Emergency Plan for AIDS Relief (PEPFAR) in 2003, established itself as a global leader in the fight against HIV/AIDS. Through PEPFAR and support for the Global Fund to Fight AIDS, Tuberculosis and Malaria, the United States helped galvanize an extraordinary global response to a single disease and mobilize donor and private-sector resources on an unprecedented scale to respond to the costly but critical task of addressing the HIV/AIDS crisis. Perhaps most important, this response demonstrated, in the face of considerable skepticism at the time, that dramatically expanding access to HIV/AIDS treatment was possible even in the world's most resource-constrained settings (IOM, 2007). The U.S. campaign against HIV/AIDS has had a historic impact and is considered among the most significant and enduring achievements of the George W. Bush administration (Stolberg, 2008).

Yet despite its substantial immediate impact, this emergency response has failed to halt or reverse the HIV/AIDS epidemic in Africa. Indeed, as outlined in the previous chapter and Appendix A, the burden of HIV/AIDS in Africa will continue to grow. As a result of continued high HIV incidence rates, the need for lifelong HIV/AIDS treatment has grown more rapidly than the ability to initiate new patients on ART. This growing burden will place ever higher demands on health care services, including an increasing number of ambulatory and hospitalized patients requiring HIV/AIDS care, an increasing number of patients requiring ART, a substantial need for additional health care workers, and a continued rise in financial and other resource requirements.

In the context of this growing burden, the United States and the global community will face significant challenges in sustaining and expanding commitments to combating HIV/AIDS in Africa. In the United States, the effects of a historic global financial crisis and a domestic deficit approaching $2 trillion will likely drive greater congressional scrutiny of spending on foreign assistance (Garrett, 2010). Moreover, the success of the U.S. HIV/AIDS effort has, ironically, increased attention to other African health challenges, which may drive competition in resource allocation among disease and health priorities. Beyond health, U.S. interests in Africa have expanded dramatically in the last decade, resulting in growing recognition of new challenges that confront development in such areas as food security, climate change, and unemployment and creating increased competition for scarce development assistance. And as the United States vies for influence in an increasingly competitive international context, it will seek new forms of engagement in Africa that provide greater political and economic leverage than traditional development and humanitarian assistance (Independent Task Force Report No. 56, 2006).

As new HIV infections continue to outstrip the world's willingness to provide ART to those in need, the costs of treatment alone will consume ever larger proportions of available resources. The combination of competing health and development demands, the rising cost burden of HIV/AIDS treatment, and continued resource constraints will force difficult choices and trade-offs for U.S. policy makers, made more politically sensitive by heightened expectations around U.S. commitments. As the largest single contributor to global HIV/AIDS resource flows to date, the United States will need to manage these choices and trade-offs in a way that does not compromise the global achievements in HIV/AIDS; advances U.S. interests; and strengthens current and future global capacities to respond to HIV/AIDS, as well as other global health challenges.

One way for the United States to accomplish these goals while addressing its own fiscal concerns is to transition to a model for long-term sustainability. This model would be one of shared responsibility with African partner states and the broader international community. By looking to African partner states to assume increasing responsibility for leadership, management, and investment of resources in HIV/AIDS, the United States would be promoting a future of self-reliance and self-sustainability. Under this shared-responsibility model, the United States would assist African partner states in developing the leadership, academic, medical, research, and other capacities necessary to assume that responsibility effectively. Implementation of this model would necessitate greater accountability and transparency in the investments being made by each African partner state. Similarly, the United States would need to take an approach grounded in realism, setting ambitious but realistic objectives for the next 10 to 15 years and placing an urgent and consistent focus on prevention of new HIV infections.

This chapter begins by describing the U.S. contributions to the global HIV/AIDS response. It next details the implications of the African HIV/AIDS burden for a variety of U.S. interests, including diplomacy, the private sector, research and academia, and foundations. The chapter then assesses the policy challenges that lie ahead for the United States in addressing these impacts and offers recommendations for moving forward in the fight against HIV/AIDS in Africa.

U.S. CONTRIBUTIONS TO THE GLOBAL HIV/AIDS RESPONSE

While it is important to be cognizant of the policy challenges that lie ahead, it is also important to acknowledge the significant accomplishments that have resulted from U.S. leadership in the global response to HIV/AIDS. In less than a decade, U.S. engagement in combating the pandemic has had a dramatic impact, particularly in Africa, the predominant focus of PEPFAR's initial phase (Independent Task Force Report No. 56, 2006; UNAIDS and WHO, 2009). Beyond the immediate human impacts, U.S. leadership has stimulated the global community and created new awareness of and support for global health among U.S. domestic actors and institutions. Finally, the U.S. response has built new partnerships in Africa and in the broader international community that ultimately strengthen the nation's standing in an increasingly competitive, multipolar global political environment (Pew Research Center, 2008; Ray, 2008).

The human impact of U.S. investments in HIV/AIDS has been profound. At the end of 2003, the year President Bush announced the PEPFAR initiative, an estimated 100,000 people, or 2 percent of those in need, were receiving ART in Africa (WHO et al., 2009). As of September 2009, more than 2.4 million people, approximately 20 percent of those in need, had access to life-saving ART because of direct bilateral PEPFAR support (PEPFAR, 2009b). Figure 3-1 shows the cumulative years of life gained through 2009 as a result of PEPFAR support for ART.

An additional 1.9 million individuals in Africa receive treatment through programs supported by the Global Fund to Fight AIDS, Tuberculosis and Malaria (Global Fund, 2010a), to which the United States is the largest national contributor. Figure 3-2 shows that 3.7 million people in low- and middle-income countries had been supported by PEPFAR and the Global Fund as of September

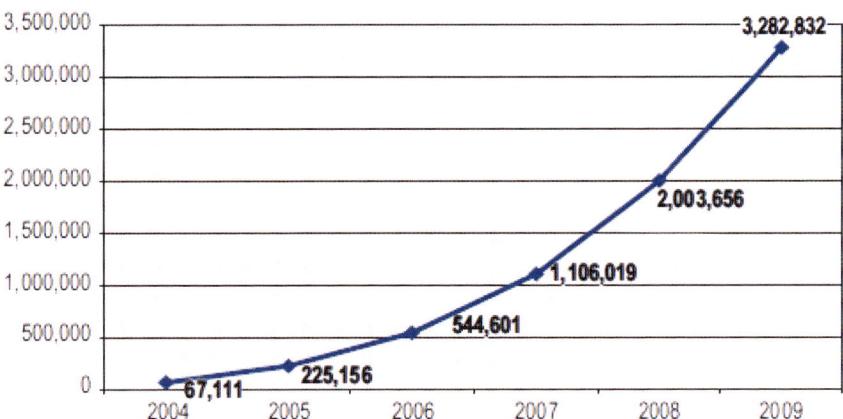

FIGURE 3-1 Cumulative years of life gained through 2009 as a result of PEPFAR support for antiretroviral therapy.
SOURCE: PEPFAR, 2009a.

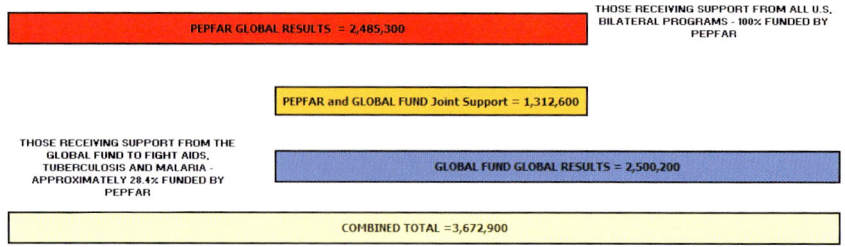

FIGURE 3-2 People receiving treatment with U.S. bilateral and multilateral support as of September 2009.
SOURCE: PEPFAR, 2010.

2009. In 2009, 6.4 million pregnant women in Africa received antenatal HIV counseling and testing because of PEPFAR, and 504,800 received antiretroviral (ARV) prophylaxis (PEPFAR, 2010). In 2009, PEPFAR gave direct HIV/AIDS and tuberculosis care and support to 6.9 million people living with HIV/AIDS and supported 3.5 million orphans and vulnerable children in Africa (PEPFAR, 2010).

At the same time, U.S. investments in responding to HIV/AIDS have advanced U.S. interests well beyond the pandemic and laid the foundation for a more comprehensive approach to public health and broader global support. U.S. leadership contributed directly to the formation of new international initiatives such as the Global Fund, with the United States providing an early $200 million in seed money, investing considerable attention in the early formation and structure of the fund (Summers, 2002) and remaining the largest single contributor to the fund since its inception. U.S. leadership has challenged other international donors to expand their investments in HIV/AIDS (see Figure 3-3) and led to the creation of numerous new public–private partnerships in the global HIV/AIDS response.

Within the United States, the PEPFAR initiative created greater public awareness of global HIV/AIDS and support for foreign aid. Beginning with the January 2002 State of the Union Address in which he first outlined the PEPFAR initiative, President Bush made combating HIV/AIDS a signature element of his foreign assistance strategy, brought home to the public through multiple trips by the President and the First Lady to African and non-African PEPFAR countries and numerous public statements and White House ceremonies highlighting the accomplishments of the initiative. Congressional travel, public speeches, and hearings on the initiative further raised the profile of global HIV/AIDS, and the focus within the U.S. government on HIV/AIDS helped fuel greater media coverage of the pandemic and the U.S. response. PEPFAR, which was the largest component of a near tripling of foreign assistance to Africa during the Bush administration (Fletcher, 2006), also garnered a robust bipartisan consensus within Congress in support of U.S. leadership; instigated a growing interest and activism among U.S.

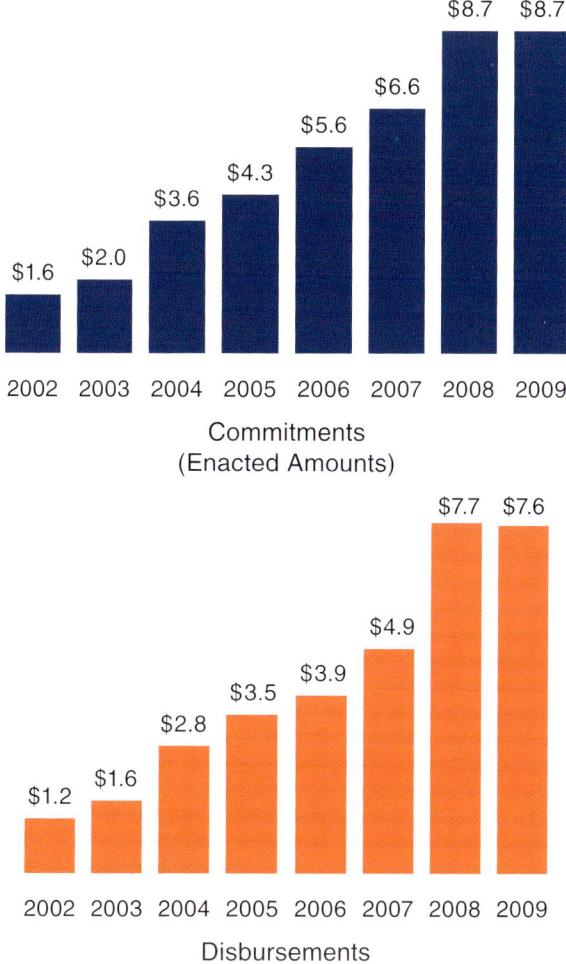

FIGURE 3-3 Steady increase in international funding for HIV/AIDS from Group of Eight (G8), European Community (EC), and other donor governments, 2002–2009 (in billions of U.S. dollars).
SOURCE: Kaiser Family Foundation, 2010.

faith-based communities with respect to development and poverty relief in Africa by opening up new areas of potential funding; and inspired new efforts by, among others, private foundations, public health researchers, political scientists, and development economists. Many of these groups brought to the forefront of U.S. leadership's attention such potentially contentious issues as how the United States plans to deal with the human, health, security, and economic implications of the projected international trends in HIV/AIDS. These new constituencies could be valuable sources of information for building a long-term strategy to combat HIV/AIDS, as well as influential bases of support for future efforts in global health.

Although the PEPFAR initiative has maintained a singular focus on HIV/AIDS, it has helped raise the profile of global health more broadly and catalyzed greater interest in the complexities of development and public health. As evidenced by adjustments to PEPFAR, new emphases in successive congressional authorizations, and the Obama administration's Global Health Initiative, U.S. interventions in HIV/AIDS through PEPFAR quickly revealed the enduring challenges of gender inequity; health infrastructure deficits; shortages of health professionals; multiple disease threats; and the intersection of public health with education, economic development, and food security. PEPFAR's early lessons have helped inform U.S. efforts going forward and have piqued the interest and commitment of a younger generation increasingly attracted to international service. Research and university partnerships have expanded, as have innovative public–private partnerships in health service delivery, training, and capacity building. These achievements will ultimately strengthen a long-term, comprehensive approach to HIV/AIDS, but also bring greater focus to the broader disease burden and structural development challenges faced by African countries.

IMPLICATIONS FOR U.S. INTERESTS

Implications for Diplomacy

PEPFAR funding and programming have engaged U.S. researchers, public health experts, technical experts, military personnel, and others with counterparts in African governments and communities in ways that simply would not have happened absent the PEPFAR platform. These interactions have impacts beyond HIV/AIDS: they build trust, strengthen a sense of shared purpose and responsibility, and foster abiding relationships that ultimately redound to U.S. interests in greater global engagement and understanding. African opinion of the United States has remained overwhelmingly positive in the last decade (Pew Research Center, 2008; Ray, 2008). Many observers attribute this goodwill to U.S. leadership and engagement in combating HIV/AIDS. While U.S. funding for HIV/AIDS treatment, which is, of necessity, a substantial long-term commitment, does not necessarily give U.S. policy makers greater leverage over recalcitrant authoritarian states in Africa (Lyman and Wittels, 2010), the linkages to individuals and communities built today may offer a basis for stronger partnerships in the future.

Finally, a less tangible but equally important outcome of U.S. global HIV/AIDS efforts has been to help rebuild the positive stature and constructive role of the United States in the world—a role that draws on international partnerships, such as those with European governments, United Nations agency heads, and African leaders, to tackle the world's most vexing transnational problems and is based on a core belief in the value of human dignity. Such leadership is all the more strategically important in a global context that is vastly different from that of 10 or 15 years ago, one in which the United States must compete with emerging powers and ideologies for alliance and influence. There is growing consensus, reiterated in the Obama administration's 2010 National Security Strategy,[1] on the need to rebuild and strengthen the elements of U.S. soft power[2] and build a "whole of government" approach—integrating the military, diplomacy, development, intelligence, and security arenas—to U.S. engagement in the world (The White House, 2010). By sustaining its commitment to the fight against HIV/AIDS and bringing the multiple elements of U.S. soft power to bear—including capacities in research, education, technology, public health, private enterprise, and philanthropic institutions—the United States has at once had an impact on the pandemic and begun to burnish its credentials as a global force for positive change.

Implications for the Private Sector

The last decade has seen a dramatic rise in private-sector engagement on HIV/AIDS, involving advocacy, philanthropic contributions, in-country programming, in-kind donations, and an array of innovative public–private partnerships (IOM, 2009a). Many companies have recognized the reputational benefits of engagement and advocacy on HIV/AIDS and have found resonance with a U.S. consumer base that is socially conscious and better informed on the scope of the pandemic.

Corporations with operations in Africa, particularly those with large employee bases, have recognized the potential impact of HIV/AIDS on their workforce—in absenteeism, productivity declines, health care expenditures, and workforce turnover—and on the broader communities in which they operate. Provision of HIV/AIDS services to employees, their families, and the communities in which they live thus serves the purposes of both corporate social responsibility and good business sense.

Through the Global Business Coalition on HIV/AIDS, Tuberculosis and Malaria (GBC), for example, corporate-sector members (such as Chevron from the United States, South Africa's Standard Bank, and nearly 200 others) align with a network built for action and achievement in the fight against infectious disease. GBC also manages the private-sector delegation to the Global Fund (GBC, 2010). Similarly, the South African Business Coalition on HIV & AIDS

---

[1] A document released by the Obama administration that lays out a strategic approach for advancing U.S. interests, including the security of the American people, a growing U.S. economy, support for our values, and an international order that can address 21st-century challenges.

[2] Soft power denotes the theory that the United States can achieve foreign policy objectives by attracting others through the legitimacy of U.S. policies and the values that underlie them, rather than through coercion with threats or payments (Nye, 2006).

(SABCOHA) coordinates a private-sector response to HIV/AIDS by empowering its members to plan for and effectively manage the impact of the epidemic in that nation. Its major projects include BizAIDS—a series of workshops with supportive materials to help micro and small companies reduce their operational risk and make them aware of the burden of HIV/AIDS—and supply chain management projects that aim to broaden the reach of private-sector HIV/AIDS initiatives (SABCOHA, 2010).

Corporate social responsibility and corporate philanthropy have brought significant resources to the global effort on HIV/AIDS, but equally important has been the rise in private–public partnerships that bring a company's core competence to bear. Companies engage in public–private partnerships for a variety of reasons, including not only corporate philanthropic objectives but also more business-driven motivations. Such partnerships can improve market access and foster partnerships and goodwill with host country governments. They can also build capacities that, while benefiting partner organizations, may serve corporate interests as well, for example, in research and development; procurement, supply chain, and other logistics management; manufacturing of pharmaceuticals; adaptation of specific technologies; laboratory building; and development of a trained and knowledgeable workforce. Ultimately, these kinds of partnerships with direct relevance to a company's business will be the most durable and sustainable, since philanthropic giving alone will be vulnerable to financial and economic fluctuations (IFC, 2008).

Pharmaceutical companies are vital to the fight against HIV/AIDS in developing new technologies, providing an adequate supply of drugs and technologies, and conducting critically needed research and development. In the early 2000s, pharmaceutical companies were a target of global HIV/AIDS activism, ultimately acquiescing to dramatic price reductions for first-line ARV drugs for the developing world. That experience may better prepare companies for future demands, but may also lead some to disinvest in research and development for products that are perceived as ultimately not serving bottom-line business interests. Already there are signs of a troubling decline in commercial investments in research and development for HIV/AIDS vaccines, microbicides, and prevention (AVAC, 2010).

As demand for affordable access to treatment increases in the future, companies will face strong downward pressure on prices for second-line therapies; new, more effective drugs; and other medical technologies. The World Trade Organization's (WTO's) Agreement on Trade Related Aspects of Intellectual Property Rights (TRIPS) includes a number of limitations and exceptions for developing countries that enable the import and manufacture of generic versions of needed drugs, although both the United States and some pharmaceutical companies have been accused at various times of retaliating against countries that choose to exercise these flexibilities (American University Washington College of Law Program on Information Justice and Intellectual Property, 2010). Moreover, as some of these exemptions for developing countries expire in 2016, tensions around intellectual property rights may increase. A number of companies have negotiated creative licensing agreements with partner states—for example, Gilead Science's arrangements with Indian and South African manufacturers to assist them in producing tenofovir while retaining patent rights—arrangements that offer hope of expanded and more sustainable access to drugs in Africa and the rest of the developing world (Bate, 2010).

Pharmaceutical companies have been strong proponents of patent protection in their attempts to protect their markets and profit margins. The result has been the perception that they place profit ahead of human welfare, a criticism that the sector has vigorously been trying to shed. Approaches to addressing this challenge include dual pricing (substantially lower prices in developing than in developed countries), voluntary licensing to developing-country generic drug manufacturers, and the creation of low-priced "generic equivalents" for low-income countries. While these approaches have increased access to affordable drugs, they have also enabled pharmaceutical companies to protect their lucrative developed-country markets and their patent provisions. In addition, pressure and support for voluntary patent pooling are rising. UNITAID, for example, announced its intention to launch a patent pool for HIV/AIDS drugs in mid-2010, an arrangement in which branded pharmaceutical companies will voluntarily waive patent rights in low-income countries in exchange for royalty fees, allowing production by local generic manufacturers while maintaining patent rights in higher-income countries. Some companies have embraced the model, although for others, questions around eligibility persist (UNITAID, 2010).

For the global effort against HIV/AIDS, it will be important that private-sector involvement and investment in new drugs and technologies be maintained (see the case example in Box 3-1). But are there adequate market signals and incentives for the development and manufacture of critically important drugs and technologies? Pharmaceutical and health technology manufacturers could help define and advocate for adequate, realistic incentive structures and advance purchasing mechanisms that would ensure investment in those drugs and technologies most relevant to the developing world. Organizations such as the Clinton Foundation and mechanisms such as UNITAID can serve as important interlocutors in these discussions.

Implications for Research and Academia

As noted, the HIV/AIDS pandemic and U.S. global efforts have attracted the attention of a younger generation increasingly interested in international service (Drain et al., 2007; IOM, 2009a,b). The last decade has seen an explosion of public and global health degree programs and multidisciplinary global health institutes at U.S. universities. A recent survey of 37 universities by the Coalition of Universities in Global Health revealed more than a doubling of the numbers

---

BOX 3-1
Building Drug Manufacturing Capacity: A Case Example

Public–private partnerships can lend themselves to building not only human resource capacity but also drug manufacturing capacity. In 1989, Merck Pharmaceuticals, Inc. signed an agreement with the Chinese Ministry of Public Health to share Merck's recombinant hepatitis B vaccine technology with two Chinese vaccine manufacturers. At the time, China had one of the highest hepatitis B rates in the world and limited production of plasma-derived hepatitis B vaccines.

Through this partnership, Merck provided China with the process design knowledge needed to produce the hepatitis B vaccine and the training needed to operate the new technology. The Chinese ministry constructed the manufacturing facility, purchased the equipment, and managed the production of the vaccine in the newly built facilities. Over a 3-year period, Chinese engineers, quality control scientists, and production supervisors trained at Merck facilities in the United States, learning the design process, assembly, and testing for the manufacturing equipment. The equipment was then shipped and installed in China, with Merck employees assisting in the reassembly.

Sixty-five percent of China's hepatitis B vaccines are now produced in these facilities, preventing more than 30 million chronic hepatitis B infections and related sequelae (Feinberg, 2010). This example of a pharmaceutical company building capacity for drug manufacturing can be applied to Africa and ART for HIV/AIDS.

---

of undergraduate, graduate, and doctoral students in global health studies in just 3 years, from 2006 to 2009. In addition, these 37 universities have a combined 302 long-term training and education projects in 97 countries around the world. Beyond the dramatic enrollment figures, the survey found that students had formed 105 global health groups—nearly three per campus (CUGH, 2009). Universities can capitalize on this burgeoning interest and broaden the interdisciplinary focus on global health and HIV/AIDS, encouraging inter- and intrauniversity collaborations and joint degree programs in public health, nursing, business, management, policy, and international affairs. Collaborations with African academic institutions, through faculty and student exchanges, distance learning, and shared curricula, can enrich both U.S. universities and African counterparts (IOM, 2005, 2009b).

U.S. academic institutions have played a key role in supporting and collaborating with African researchers to make substantial contributions to the generation of new knowledge, especially in the areas of clinical and public health research on HIV/AIDS. U.S.–African research partnerships are well established and have a long track record of building local capacity to conduct research. Most notable among these initiatives is the Fogarty AIDS International Training and

Research Program, which provides funds for both U.S. partner institutions and in-country institutions with a view to long-term capacity building and increased South–South collaboration.[3] Such programs need to be expanded to more African countries as they help address, and in some instances reverse, the brain drain because of their high in-country retention rates.

At another level, strengthening of research capacity needs to extend beyond the training of individual researchers to create academically vibrant and sustainable research institutions in Africa. There are many examples of U.S. institutions creating world-class research institutes in Africa, most of which are self-sustaining with strong in-country leadership. Most notable among these are the Infectious Diseases Institute (IDI) in Uganda; the University of California, San Francisco–University of Zimbabwe (UCSF-UZ) collaboration in Zimbabwe; and the Centre for the AIDS Programme of Research in South Africa (CAPRISA). In addition, philanthropies such as the Doris Duke Charitable Foundation and the Howard Hughes Medical Institute have made substantial investments in creating major new basic science and clinical research institutes with long-term secure funding. Such long-term investments take the role of the United States in research capacity building one step further; they are strengthening institutional capacity and core resources such as libraries and access to scientific journals, building critical mass, helping to alleviate the brain drain, and creating capacity for high-quality in-country research training.

Since Africa is the region of the world most affected by HIV/AIDS, it is also the region with the greatest potential to make significant contributions to new breakthroughs in HIV/AIDS prevention and treatment. For example, Africa has contributed critically important HIV prevention strategies, such as the use of nevirapine and exclusive breastfeeding to reduce mother-to-child transmission of HIV, circumcision for the prevention of HIV in men, and topical ARV agents for HIV prevention in women. The development of these strategies was made possible by the long-term investments of the U.S. government in building clinical trial capacity in Africa. This capacity-building process occurred over decades, largely through clinical trial networks sponsored by the National Institutes of Health (NIH), which evolved from initial partnership arrangements led almost solely by U.S. investigators to the current model of partnerships of equals involving joint U.S.–African leadership. Chapter 5 provides a thorough discussion of capacity-building partnerships, including twinning, and offers recommendations for the academic sectors in the United States and Africa.

---

[3] South–South collaborations involve a horizontal relationship between two or more developing countries in which technical assistance in HIV/AIDS prevention, treatment, and care is exchanged through visits, training, and ongoing communication (AIHA, 2005).

Implications for Foundations

Addressing the HIV/AIDS epidemic in Africa speaks to the core interest and mission of a large number of U.S. philanthropies—that is, contributing to a global public good and improving the lives of those most in need. U.S. foundations have been a major force in mobilizing responses and resources for the fight against HIV/AIDS. In 2008 they provided $618 million for programming related specifically to global HIV/AIDS, 36 percent of which targeted east and southern Africa (Funders Concerned About AIDS, 2009). The Bill & Melinda Gates Foundation accounted for about 59 percent of philanthropic funding in 2008, and such funding is increasingly concentrated among a relatively small number of organizations (Funders Concerned About AIDS, 2009). Large foundations that bring significant financial resources to bear can play an important role in protecting core commitments in uncertain political or financial times.

Beyond resource mobilization, foundations have a unique role to play in complementing the efforts of governments and multilateral institutions. Political independence gives them flexibility and the ability to innovate and take risks and to support interventions and programming in areas less likely than others to generate broad-based political support. There is tremendous variety across U.S. philanthropic organizations in objectives, time frames, and strategies, and this diversity is an additional asset in building a long-term, sustainable response to HIV/AIDS. Relatively new foundations, such as the Bill & Melinda Gates Foundation, have emphasized innovation (The Bill & Melinda Gates Foundation, 2010), pioneering efforts that may entail higher risk than most government programming is willing or able to bear. The Gates Foundation has played a vital role in sustaining commitment to HIV/AIDS vaccine and prevention research (AVAC, 2010) and has been the largest private contributor to the Global Fund (Global Fund, 2010c). It has had a strong political voice and helped catalyze efforts of a host of nongovernmental organizations in advocacy, prevention, and research. The Clinton Foundation, through the Clinton Health Access Initiative, has undertaken an innovative business-oriented approach, working with generic pharmaceutical companies in international efforts to reduce the price of drugs and medical technologies for low-income countries, as well as engaging in service delivery, training, and health policy assistance (Clinton Foundation, 2010). These and similar foundations have generated new knowledge and lessons learned; they have the ability to be nimble and adaptive and to reach communities and address issues that are politically marginalized or controversial.

On the other hand, long-standing U.S. foundations—such as the Ford Foundation, the Carnegie Corporation of New York, the John D. and Catherine T. MacArthur Foundation, the Rockefeller Foundation, the William and Flora Hewlett Foundation, and the Africa America Institute—have remarkable track records in building research, academic, and leadership capacity through sustained, long-term engagement. The mechanisms they have used include fellowships, partnerships, and scholarships, the kinds of investments that do not yield quick returns but are critical in building the longer-term capacities that will be needed to address HIV/AIDS in coming generations.

Collaboration and communication among diverse U.S.-based foundations will be valuable in harnessing the strengths of each, sharing best practices and lessons learned, and identifying potential areas of need or neglect. Funders Concerned About AIDS (FCAA), which comprises some 1,500 private philanthropic organizations focused on HIV/AIDS, has helped play this role, providing information and technical advice to foundations and tracking trend lines in funding and programming for HIV/AIDS across U.S. philanthropies (Funders Concerned About AIDS, 2010).

The ability of philanthropic organizations to operate outside the control of donor and recipient governments is a benefit, although this independence does come with potential risks, particularly when significant resource flows are involved. Bringing disproportionate resources and innovation to bear on a problem of interest to a particular philanthropy but outside a national government's strategic plan can potentially have distorting effects by drawing essential personnel and resources away from the host country's priority challenges. Further, as efficiency of programming and rationalizing of multiple resource flows become increasingly important, foundations working in country will want to ensure that their efforts are aligned with or complementary to national strategies.

ADDRESSING THE IMPACTS ON U.S. INTERESTS

PEPFAR was born of an exceptional moment of international consensus around HIV/AIDS, propelled by a sense of urgency and opportunity. Today, 29 years into the pandemic and a decade after significant mobilization of the international community began, U.S. leadership in combating HIV/AIDS remains essential. In fact, such leadership is needed now more than ever, as the response to the pandemic needs to be transformed to meet the long-term challenge.

Building a Long-Term Approach to a Chronic Emergency

Among the greatest challenges will be the difficulty of maintaining a sense of urgency and focus on HIV/AIDS while responding to critics eager to move the U.S. global commitment away from such a strong emphasis on a single disease. As suggested earlier, as the initial impetus and sense of urgency for U.S. engagement on HIV/AIDS subside, U.S. policy makers will likely seek to take on new global and development challenges, and domestic constituencies and African partners will similarly press for attention and funding for competing health and development priorities. Yet HIV/AIDS remains a grave and immediate threat that puts millions of lives in jeopardy and will be an ongoing emergency for many decades to come, especially in Africa (see Chapter 2 and Appendix A).

The epidemic in the region is thus a crisis that requires an emergency response but at the same time the forethought, planning, and sustained commitment of a long-term development intervention (Whiteside and Whalley, 2007). If incidence rates do not slow significantly in the next decade, the ever-increasing demand for access to ART will threaten to overwhelm the human, institutional, and resource capacities currently available to African states and their partners. Accordingly, the international community must focus now on preventive measures and invest far greater effort in strategically building the human and institutional capacities needed to manage the epidemic in a sustainable way.

Moving beyond short-term strategies on HIV/AIDS will challenge U.S. policy makers, legislators (appropriators in particular), and the U.S. public, all of whom are eager to see quick, tangible returns on investments made (Feingold, 2007; Oomman et al., 2007; Ward, 2007). PEPFAR garnered strong bipartisan domestic support largely because it was presented as an emergency intervention and set hard targets for prevention, treatment, and care on which future funding would be predicated. Among the PEPFAR targets, expanding access to treatment has been the least difficult to measure and has had the most dramatic, immediate, and visible impact. Some have termed this rejuvenation of a community through the infusion of ART the "Lazarus" effect. This achievement has served as a powerful incentive for U.S. policy makers, who are able to see dramatic proof of the impacts of U.S. investments. More diffuse efforts in prevention, care, health system strengthening, and capacity building—critical areas for future success—have proven more difficult to measure and less immediately visible (Accordia Global Health Foundation, 2010), and thus they are potentially less likely to generate continued congressional enthusiasm. The full dividends from investments in education, training, and institution building likely will not be felt for 10 to 15 years, a considerably longer time horizon than that which typically preoccupies U.S. policy makers. In the fight against HIV/AIDS, as in development assistance more broadly, the U.S. Congress must be convinced to look beyond annual targets and undertake the longer-term commitments required for a sustained impact. To this end, the U.S. administration must forge a longer-term vision on HIV/AIDS, one that sets ambitious but realistic objectives over the next 15 years and that gives Congress and the U.S. public a sustained sense of purpose and direction for long-term U.S. investments in HIV/AIDS, as well as greater appreciation of how these investments will shape future outcomes.

Moving Toward Shared Responsibility

As noted earlier, a central feature of a long-term, sustainable approach is shared responsibility, with African partner governments assuming increasing responsibility for the mustering and management of resources for national HIV/AIDS strategies. If the United States is to sustain a long-term financial commitment to combating HIV/AIDS during a fiscal crisis, Congress and U.S. taxpayers will likely demand greater assurance that the recipients of the funding are equally engaged both in mobilizing domestic resources and in ensuring efficiency and accountability in their use. At the same time, however, managing this transition to shared responsibility and striking the appropriate balance may prove politically sensitive.

U.S. leadership to date has created an expectation of continued rapid expansion of HIV/AIDS funding among recipient governments, the international community, and domestic constituencies focused on HIV/AIDS. These expectations may prove politically damaging if the United States is perceived as reneging on commitments or unilaterally disengaging through a strategy of "country ownership." Domestic and international activists were quick to criticize the Obama administration's slowdown in funding increases for HIV/AIDS, even in the aftermath of the worst domestic economic recession in a century (AHF, 2010; Tutu, 2010; Voice of America, 2010).

The burden of expectation will be particularly acute with respect to U.S. support for treatment. Today, the United States supports the provision of ART to some 2.4 million people in need globally, and the Obama administration has promised to extend that commitment to 4 million people by 2014 (Office of the Global AIDS Coordinator, 2009). This commitment, as well as the 2005 Group of Eight (G8) commitment to achieving "as close as possible" universal access to HIV treatment by 2010 (International AIDS Society, 2010), has created a general expectation on the part of recipients and partner governments that U.S. support for treatment can continue and expand as the number of those in need of ART increases. This expectation puts U.S. policy makers in a precarious position. They cannot in good conscience withdraw support from individuals who have accessed ART through U.S. intervention. As a result, support for ART has taken on attributes of an entitlement program, which cannot, for ethical and political reasons, easily be scaled down (Over, 2008). If the rate of expanded access to ART decreases, the United States may face popular resentment and diplomatic repercussions from partner governments. Recent shortages of ARV drugs in Uganda in early 2010, attributed to the United States withholding resources, generated headlines highly critical of the U.S. administration and linking U.S. budget decisions to heartbreaking stories of patients turned away from ART clinics (McNeil, 2010; Zakumumpa, 2010).

If the gap between treatment needs and available resources increases, difficult questions will inevitably arise about how to prioritize access to ART, with individual lives hanging in the balance. Already, the Office of the Global AIDS Coordinator has indicated that preference will be given to pregnant women, tuberculosis patients, and individuals with extremely low CD4 cell counts (Goosby, 2010). The merits of this or any particular approach aside, the larger question will inevitably arise of how these decisions are made and who has the authority to make them. The United States will not serve its interests by entangling itself in complex ethical questions that are more legitimately answered within recipient states (see Chapter 6 for a more thorough discussion of the need for ethical decision-making capacity in African communities).

Although a shift to greater shared responsibility with African partner governments in the next decade is most desirable, it will not easily be accomplished in all countries. First, the question arises of whether partner states will be ready and willing to assume this role. To date, little scrutiny and expectation have been focused on African governments themselves in prioritizing or mobilizing resources for HIV/AIDS. Few African countries have come close to meeting commitments made at the Abuja summit in 2002, at which heads of state pledged to allocate 15 percent of their national budgets to the health sector. On a continental level, average general government expenditures on health as a percentage of total government expenditures rose marginally from 8.8 percent in 2001 to 9.0 percent in 2007 (the last full year for which data are available), although three countries—Djibouti, Botswana, and Rwanda—attained the target in 2007 (Global Fund, 2010d).

For most countries, external resources constitute a significant proportion of total health expenditures (the continental average in Africa rose from 15.3 percent in 2002 to 20.1 percent in 2006, with 14 countries at more than 30 percent). Many African countries remain highly dependent on external assistance for health resources (Global Fund, 2010d). In some countries, in fact, there is troubling evidence that donor assistance for health has had a negative effect on domestic government spending on health (Lu et al., 2010). Further, African partner countries vary widely with respect to the political will to assume a stronger leadership role and to develop strategic and planning capacity, management and implementation capacity, and institutional infrastructure and resources.

The question also arises of whether U.S. policy makers will be prepared to cede significant control over funding flows and allow for flexibility in meeting partner-driven, rather than U.S.-driven, priorities. The dominant role of U.S. funding in individual countries' HIV/AIDS budgets has meant that in many cases, congressional earmarks and U.S. priorities drive national responses in recipient countries. And while the Office of the Global AIDS Coordinator has placed increasing emphasis on the notion of "country ownership," it is not yet clear whether the United States, and in particular the Congress, will be prepared to act on this notion with respect to resource management and allocation.

In 2008, PEPFAR established the concept of "Partnership Frameworks"—nonbinding agreements intended as "joint strategic planning documents that outline the goals and objectives to be achieved and the commitments and contributions expected of all participating Framework members" (Office of the Global AIDS Coordinator, 2008). This approach is a strong and positive step toward clarifying the respective roles of the United States and its partners within a model of increasingly shared responsibility. Nonetheless, as resource requirements, the need for efficiency, and expectations for greater partner country investment mount, a more binding form of written agreement or contract would provide strong incentives for effective and accountable partner-country governance and investment. It would also spell out U.S. obligations and commitments in a more reliable and predictable way that would facilitate future planning by host country governments. This model would resemble the compact model of the U.S. Millennium Challenge Account (MCA), which, based on strong positive indicators in the areas of good governance, economic freedom, and investments in their citizens, gives partner countries far greater control over planning, allocation, and management for large-scale, 5-year grants (MCC, 2010).

Because African countries fall along a broad continuum in terms of their capacity to take on "full ownership," the shared-responsibility paradigm is intended to provide incentives to move toward greater ownership and help give African nations the capacities to do so. As with the MCA, countries with demonstrated political will, an emphasis on prevention, and efficient, transparent health management would receive stronger financial commitments with less control, oversight, or intervention from the United States. This approach would move the United States more in the direction of providing direct budget support. If African countries did not maintain their commitment to the binding aspects of the contract, the agreement would require a renegotiation. For the lowest-income, less-capable countries in Africa with weak leadership around HIV/AIDS, the contract model should incorporate incentives to improve their performance in order to receive increased financial support. In their relationship with these less equipped countries, the United States and other donors should play a larger role in the capacity-building aspects of the shared-responsibility paradigm, including leadership and infrastructure development, and should maintain strict oversight of budgetary support. Given the projected burden of HIV/AIDS in the coming decades, support from international donors today can help build the infrastructure, political will, and institutional and human resource capacity that African nations will need to address their own country-specific HIV/AIDS needs and priorities in 2020 and beyond.

The following are examples of what the United States and other partner governments might include as essential or "nonnegotiable" elements of such a contract relating to African government responsibilities:

- sustained political leadership on HIV/AIDS;
- commitment to human rights and an evidence-based national response to the epidemic;
- a strong focus and voice on HIV/AIDS prevention; and
- transparent, efficient, and accountable procedures for the use of both country-level and donor resources.

Those countries deemed as lacking these essential elements would not qualify for elevated levels of financing or a contract model ceding greater control to the African partner government.

The committee acknowledges that the achievement of these contract responsibilities may take time. Nevertheless, the United States should immediately make clear that it will become more selective with respect to its development partners. As less restrictive approaches to these types of institutional relationships have not succeeded in the past, it is the committee's best judgment that binding contracts—in which the United States would cut back on funding in those countries that lagged in taking the path toward shared responsibility—are worth trying in the future.

Making Prevention a Priority

The greatest challenge to U.S. policy is the continued expansion of the epidemic in Africa. Today, incidence rates remain at alarmingly high levels, outstripping expanded access to treatment by a ratio of 5 to 2—for every two people accessing ART for the first time, an estimated five people are newly infected (see Chapter 2 for a discussion of the treatment gap and associated resource requirements).

The many achievements of the U.S. global HIV/AIDS response—and indeed the global community's remarkable mobilization around the disease—are profoundly at risk if this trajectory persists. Yet despite these alarming statistics, support for prevention has been among the more politically divisive issues within the Congress, with ideological sensitivities focusing on condom promotion, sex education, outreach to commercial sex workers, and injecting drug use. Should new infections in Africa continue to outstrip access to treatment, by 2020 the costs of providing treatment will far exceed the international community's capacity and will to mobilize adequate resources. This reality must be the central driver of any future strategy on HIV/AIDS. Failure to reduce incidence rates will make the goal of universal access to treatment impossible and will result in increasingly difficult decisions about complex trade-offs and political choices in the coming decade and beyond (see Chapter 2).

Chapter 2 underscores the importance of acting now to shape outcomes that will be apparent only in the long term. Failure to act decisively on HIV/AIDS prevention now will result in an even bleaker situation in 2020 in terms of the ever-growing need and demand for treatment resources. Prevention works best when interventions are selected on the basis of knowledge of the risks and drivers of the epidemic and when they are implemented appropriately and to scale. To this end, a better balance must be struck in the allocation of effort and resources to prevention and treatment (Independent Task Force Report No. 56, 2006; UNAIDS and WHO, 2009). The overlap between the two is significant (see Chapter 2) but not absolute, and in a context of finite resources and the present fiscal situation in the United States, trade-offs in resource allocation will most certainly be necessary. However, attaining the optimum balance between treatment and prevention will likely be a politically complex issue, as saving lives through expansion of ART is the highly visible and pressing need.

Given this difficult challenge, it is important not to lose sight of the value of treatment efforts already under way while strengthening prevention messages and activities. Evidence of successes in HIV/AIDS prevention is growing; for example, the drop in new HIV infections among children between 2001 and 2009 suggests that the increase in coverage for services to prevent mother-to-child transmission of HIV is saving lives (UNAIDS, 2010).

Engaging the World: Leveraging Multilateral Assets

In today's global political context, in which the United States must increase its reliance on global alliances and partnerships, strengthening and working through multilateral mechanisms are of increasing strategic importance, a point underscored in President Obama's 2010 National Security Strategy (The White House, 2010). Accordingly, the United States will want to ensure continued international engagement on HIV/AIDS and leverage the full range of capabilities and resources that the broader global community can bring to bear.

Multilateral forums and institutions have been an important component of U.S. engagement on HIV/AIDS. They have been a strong asset for U.S. leadership in building international consensus, mobilizing resources and attention, coordinating global efforts, and creating and strengthening international institutions dedicated to global health and the fight against infectious disease. The Clinton administration's engagement in the 2000 United Nations (UN) Security Council Session on HIV/AIDS in Africa, which declared HIV in Africa a threat to security (Gore, 2000), and participation in the UN General Assembly Special Session on HIV/AIDS in 2001 (UNGASS, 2001), for example, are considered watershed events in bringing greater international attention and urgency to the HIV/AIDS pandemic. Support for UNAIDS has allowed that organization to aggregate and communicate data on the pandemic effectively and to help ensure coordination and complementarity of international efforts at the country level.

The U.S. voice at successive G8 summit meetings has helped generate significant resource commitments from G8 members in support of HIV/AIDS endeavors. Mechanisms such as UNITAID, which pursues price reductions for drugs and medical technologies, offer models for innovative financing and market incentives that complement U.S. bilateral funding flows. Today, as the Group of Twenty (G20) gains global traction, the United States should seek to broaden discussions on global health and encourage continued attention to HIV/AIDS. It should make a particular effort to engage emerging economic powers, including China, India, Russia, and Brazil, both in formulating multilateral strategies on HIV/AIDS and in strengthening human resource– and capacity-building collaborations within South–South partnerships.

Perhaps most important in the multilateral arena, early U.S. support for the Global Fund helped initiate and sustain a new model of international financial support that is driven by country-level plans, priorities, and decision making (Global Fund, 2010b). How best to strike an appropriate balance between U.S. bilateral commitments and commitments channeled through multilateral mechanisms such as the Global Fund has been the source of ongoing domestic debate. Both approaches have their merits and shortcomings.

Bilateral programming has allowed the United States to channel resources quickly to recipient countries; realize quick returns on short-term investments; and retain close control, oversight, and accountability in U.S. funding flows. The pressure to see quick results led to an early tendency by PEPFAR implementers to seek to bypass weak, inefficient systems in recipient countries. PEPFAR's decision to initially operate independently of existing mechanisms was key to making things happen quickly in partner organizations (as centralizing and coordinating slows down operations). In this sense, the approach was pragmatic and timely, but it did undermine host countries' abilities to attain greater coordination. For this reason, bilateral programs have been criticized for creating parallel procurement and service delivery systems, for failing to integrate fully with recipient country priorities, and for tending toward short-term strategies that do not necessarily give priority to capacity building or sustainability.

The Global Fund model, on the other hand, ensures that funding flows are more clearly aligned with country priorities as determined by a multisectoral Country Coordinating Mechanism; that recipients enjoy greater flexibility in using resources for long-term approaches and system strengthening; and that more responsibility is placed with host countries for planning, management, and institutional capacity to oversee and account for health resources. This model also has been criticized, however, for such reasons as slow disbursements of funding, reliance on in-country capacities that are overly weak or politicized, and laborious bureaucratic processes.

No doubt both U.S. bilateral efforts and the Global Fund will require adjustments as the HIV/AIDS pandemic and country capacities evolve. By analyzing these efforts over the coming decade, the United States could capitalize on the positive aspects of both models; the committee calls for drawing on the best of both approaches. For example, as a recipient country's capacity for delivery, management, and oversight of interventions becomes more robust, the United States may want to shift away from bilateral interventions to multilateral funding mechanisms. The committee does not expect this shift to occur overnight, but sees its progressive realization as a potentially important long-term goal of the proposed shared-responsibility model. The U.S. effort can help remedy inadequate infrastructure and systems only if the host country itself has the will to do so.

Striving for Integration and Efficiency

U.S. commitments to combating HIV/AIDS, and in particular the growing costs associated with expanded provision of treatment, may ultimately limit U.S. flexibility and ability to address the health and development priorities articulated by African partner states. Since 2001, HIV/AIDS has dominated U.S. global health funding. Critical investments in family planning, in maternal-child health, and in early childhood diseases have not seen increases commensurate with those in HIV/AIDS services, although they face devastating challenges in virtually every African state. The Obama administration's expanded Global Health Initiative budget for 2010 includes significant increases in family planning and maternal-child health, but PEPFAR programming is expected to make up some 77 percent of overall funding flows (Kaiser Family Foundation, 2009).

Accusations of "AIDS exceptionalism" may intensify, especially if expenditures on ARV drugs consume an ever larger proportion of U.S. global health spending. Policy makers may face increasing pressure from U.S domestic interests, donor partners, and African partner governments to address more directly health priorities beyond HIV/AIDS and to support multipurpose investments in health system strengthening.[4] In a world of finite financial resources, policy makers must confront difficult trade-offs, including that between focusing on life-prolonging ARV drug purchases and envisioning HIV/AIDS in a broader context of pressing and equally devastating disease challenges.

Just as striking the right balance between prevention and treatment efforts will be difficult for governments, striking the appropriate balance between funding for HIV/AIDS and other diseases will be an ongoing and sensitive political challenge. Identifying and strengthening synergies between HIV/AIDS interventions and other health objectives may alleviate some of this difficulty. To this end, implementers on the ground might proactively seek opportunities for integration of HIV/AIDS services and capacities with other disease and development interventions. Funders could help as well by identifying and developing approaches that better integrate HIV/AIDS interventions with other critical health priorities. For the U.S. government, this might mean better integration of global health efforts and improved alignment with host country priorities. By giving greater priority to those interventions that build enduring health care capacity, the United States can enable African partners to manage the multiple challenges their citizens confront.

An even broader challenge will be balancing HIV/AIDS and other health interventions with other forms of U.S. development assistance. In the course of the last decade, Africa has moved more firmly into the mainstream of U.S. policy with an expansion of U.S. interests and investments; a changing notion of what

---

[4] An assessment of positive, negative, or neutral spillover effects of HIV/AIDS-targeted programs on health systems is discussed in Chapter 4.

constitutes security; and greater competition for influence and alliance in an increasingly globalized, multipolar international context. Engagement on HIV/ AIDS has been an important component of expanded U.S. relations with Africa, but only one of many strands of additional attention and concern. Support for HIV/AIDS programming represents a growing proportion of U.S. development assistance to Africa overall. In many African countries, HIV/AIDS and other health funding is by far the largest component of U.S. assistance. In Nigeria, HIV/ AIDS constitutes 77 percent of U.S. State Department/U.S. Agency for International Development (USAID) assistance, and overall health programming constitutes 89 percent of assistance (USAID, 2009b); in Rwanda, the corresponding proportions are 60 percent and 79 percent (USAID, 2009c); in Kenya, 77 percent and 88 percent (USAID, 2009a); and in Uganda, 64 percent and 83 percent (USAID, 2009d).[5] Investments in agriculture, in education, and in democracy and governance are dwarfed by HIV/AIDS funding, although each of those areas intersects in significant ways with public health and is viewed by many African governments as an important development priority in its own right. Further, expanded investments in HIV/AIDS and health will ultimately yield diminishing marginal returns if other critical developmental priorities—employment, food security, economic growth, education, and water and sanitation—remain unaddressed. Domestic critics may argue that U.S. efforts in international development are too heavily skewed toward HIV/AIDS and that areas of pressing international and foreign policy concern are being neglected.

HIV/AIDS interventions, some observers argue, may be popular among African partner countries, but they do not necessarily lead to greater leverage or influence (Lyman and Wittels, 2010). U.S. policy makers are understandably reluctant to use support for HIV/AIDS services or other forms of humanitarian assistance as a political bargaining chip. But the domination of HIV/AIDS within U.S. foreign assistance flows means there is little room for other forms of engagement that might provide that leverage. The 2010 National Security Strategy promises that "the United States will work to remain an attractive and influential partner by ensuring that African priorities such as infrastructure development, improving reliable access to power, and increased trade and investment remain high on our agenda" (The White House, 2010). Similarly, the administration has announced global food security as a top priority, with President Obama promising $3.5 billion to strengthen food security and enlisting the G8 to give greater priority to assisting poor farmers (Baker and Dugger, 2009; Council on Foreign Relations, 2009). A renewed focus on agricultural development through the Feed the Future initiative was welcomed by development experts and African leaders alike, who have seen investment in agricultural development fall from a high of 18 percent of official development assistance in 1979 to 3.5 percent in 2004 (World Bank, 2008). But unless the overall flow of U.S. assistance increases dra-

---

[5] Percentages calculated using fiscal year 2010 estimates.

matically, there will be little room for these new initiatives—or for other major initiatives not yet envisioned—given current commitments to PEPFAR and global health. U.S. support for HIV/AIDS assistance to Africa is authorized primarily by the 1961 Foreign Assistance Act as well as the PEPFAR legislation, which was reauthorized in 2008 for an additional 5 years.[6] The 1961 Foreign Assistance Act was last reauthorized in 2002, and the Congress is currently designing new legislation to update the act. This overhaul offers an opportunity to incorporate some of the steps toward shared responsibility that are described in this report.

RECOMMENDATIONS

Recommendation 3-1[7]: *Emphasize a new contract approach that incentivizes shared responsibility.* The Office of the Global AIDS Coordinator should emphasize, develop, and implement a more binding, negotiated contract approach at the country level. The contract should incentivize shared responsibility whereby additive donor resources are provided to a large extent as matching funds for partner countries' investments of their own domestic resources in health. Such matching funds should not be a uniform ratio; rather, the ratio should vary based on each African partner's ability to contribute.

Recommendation 3-2: *Develop a U.S. roadmap for HIV/AIDS in 2020.* The White House and the Office of the Global AIDS Coordinator should develop a U.S. roadmap for HIV/AIDS in 2020 incorporating a model of U.S.–African shared responsibility that makes prevention a priority and balances bilateral and multilateral funding. The roadmap should:

- Give priority to prevention as a central tenet of a sustainable long-term response to the HIV/AIDS epidemic. To this end, steps should be taken to:
    - strengthen country-level surveillance and monitoring of the epidemic to ensure adequate and reliable data with which to estimate incidence rates (see Recommendation 2-1);
    - encourage the UNAIDS-recommended approach of targeted prevention strategies tailored to in-country priority populations, applying evidence-based public health approaches;
    - increase access to and coverage of synergistic combinations of known effective prevention technologies; and
    - expand research and investments in new prevention technologies.

---

[6] *Tom Lantos and Henry J. Hyde United States Global Leadership against HIV/AIDS, Tuberculosis, and Malaria Reauthorization Act of 2008*, Public Law 110-293 (July 30, 2008).

[7] See counterpart Recommendation 4-3 directed to African countries (Chapter 4).

- Strike an optimal balance between bilateral and multilateral mechanisms for HIV/AIDS funding. The United States should seek to capitalize on the strategic complementarity of bilateral and multilateral funding flows and engagement and work to strengthen multilateral institutions toward that end. U.S. policy makers should encourage greater involvement of emerging economic powers, including Brazil, China, Russia, and India, in international forums and activities on HIV/AIDS and in strengthening of South–South collaborations addressing the epidemic.

Recommendation 3-3: *Integrate health and development.* Congress should support greater integration of U.S.-funded HIV/AIDS interventions with broader U.S. global health initiatives and African countries' comprehensive development plans. As Congress contemplates an overhaul of the U.S. Foreign Assistance Act, it should seek to encourage greater flexibility in development funding to ensure that assistance for both health and development meets recipient country priorities.

REFERENCES

Accordia Global Health Foundation. 2010. *Return on investment: The long-term impact of building healthcare capacity in Africa.* Washington, DC: Accordia Global Health Foundation.

AHF (AIDS Healthcare Foundation). 2010. *AHF to roll out "Who's better on AIDS?" Obama/Bush comparison ad campaign in DC.* http://www.aidshealth.org/news/press-releases/ahf-president-obama-fails.html (accessed May 20, 2010).

AIHA (American International Health Alliance). 2005. *HIV/AIDS twinning center frequently asked questions.* http://www.twinningagainstaids.org/faq.html (accessed November 2, 2009).

American University Washington College of Law Program on Information Justice and Intellectual Property. 2010. Complaint to UN special rapporteur on the right to health, July 19, 2010.

AVAC: Global Advocacy for HIV Prevention. 2010. *AVAC report 2010: Turning the page.* New York: AVAC.

Baker, B., and C. Dugger. 2009. Obama enlists major powers to aid poor farmers with $15 billion. *The New York Times.*

Bate, R. 2010. Solving an innovator's dilemma. *The American: Journal of the American Enterprise Institute.* http://www.american.com/archive/2010/may/solving-an-innovators-dilemma (accessed May 20, 2010).

The Bill & Melinda Gates Foundation. 2010. *Overview: The Gates Foundation's HIV strategy.* http://www.gatesfoundation.org/hivaids/Documents/hiv-strategy-overview.pdf (accessed September 7, 2010).

Clinton Foundation. 2010. *Why global health? Our approach.* http://www.clintonfoundation.org/what-we-do/clinton-health-access-initiative/our-approach (accessed September 7, 2010).

CUGH (Consortium of Universities for Global Health). 2009. *Saving lives: Universities transforming global health.* San Francisco, CA: CUGH.

Council on Foreign Relations. 2009. *Obama's food security initiative in Africa.* http://www.cfr.org/publication/20020/obamas_food_security_initiative_in_africa.html (accessed October 6, 2010).

Drain, P. K., A. Primack, D. D. Hunt, W. W. Fawzi, K. K. Holmes, and P. Gardner. 2007. Global health in medical education: A call for more training and opportunities. *Academic Medicine* 82(3):226-230.

Feinberg, M. 2010 (unpublished). *Public-private partnerships addressing diseases of the developing world: Lessons learned; current challenges; future opportunities.* Merck & Co. Inc.

Feingold, R. 2007. Remarks of U.S. Senator Russ Feingold on priorities for PEPFAR reauthorization.

Fletcher, M. 2006. Bush has quietly tripled aid to Africa. *The Washington Post.*

Funders Concerned About AIDS. 2009. *U.S. philanthropic support to address HIV/AIDS in 2008.* Brooklyn, NY: Funders Concerned About AIDS.

———. 2010. *Mission & vision.* http://www.fcaaids.org/AboutFCAA/MissionVision/tabid/171/Default.aspx (accessed August 26, 2010).

Garrett, L. 2010. *The debate over foreign aid.* Washington, DC: Council on Foreign Relations.

GBC (Global Business Coalition on HIV/AIDS Tuberculosis and Malaria). 2010. *Collaboration, coordination and collective action that will end disease faster.* http://www.gbcimpact.org/about-gbc (accessed September 24, 2010).

Global Fund. 2010a. *The Global Fund 2010: Innovation and impact.* Geneva: Global Fund.

———. 2010b. *How the Global Fund works.* http://www.theglobalfund.org/en/how/?lang=en (accessed September 7, 2010).

———. 2010c. *Partnering for global health: The Global Fund and the private sector.* Geneva: Global Fund.

———. 2010d. *Trends in development assistance and domestic financing for health in implementing countries.* Geneva: Global Fund.

Goosby, E. 2010. Presentation to IOM committee on envisioning a strategy to prepare for the long-term burden of HIV/AIDS: African needs and U.S. interests, Pretoria, South Africa, April 12, 2010.

Gore, A. 2000. Remarks as prepared for delivery by Vice President Al Gore: UN security council session on AIDS in Africa. Paper read at UN Security Council Session on HIV/AIDS in Africa.

IFC (International Finance Corporation). 2008. *Business of health in Africa: Partnering with the private sector to improve people's lives.* Washington, DC: IFC.

Independent Task Force Report No. 56. 2006. *More than humanitarianism: A strategic U.S. approach toward Africa.* New York: Council on Foreign Relations, Inc.

International AIDS Society. 2010. *IAS urges G8 to follow through on prior commitment to universal access to HIV prevention, treatment and care by 2010 as part of new maternal and child health initiative.* http://www.iasociety.org/Default.aspx?pageId=393 (accessed October 21, 2010).

IOM (Institute of Medicine). 2005. *Healers abroad: Americans responding to the human resource crisis in HIV/AIDS.* Washington, DC: The National Academies Press.

———. 2007. *PEPFAR implementation: Progress and promise.* Washington, DC: The National Academies Press.

———. 2009a. *The U.S. commitment to global health: Recommendations for the new administration.* Washington, DC: The National Academies Press.

———. 2009b. *The U.S. commitment to global health: Recommendations for the public and private sectors.* Edited by P. Subramanian. Washington, DC: The National Academies Press.

Kaiser Family Foundation. 2009. *Fact sheet: The U.S. President's Emergency Plan for AIDS Relief (PEPFAR).* Washington, DC: Kaiser Family Foundation.

———. 2010. *International AIDS assistance: Trends in G8/EC and other donor government assistance, 2002-2009.* Washington, DC: Kaiser Family Foundation.

Lu, C., M. T. Schneider, P. O. Gubbins, K. Leach-Kemon, D. T. Jamison, and C. J. Murray. 2010. Public financing of health in developing countries: A cross-national systematic analysis. *The Lancet* 375(9723):1375-1387.

Lyman, P. N., and S. B. Wittels. 2010. No good deed goes unpunished. *Foreign Affairs* 89(4):74-84.

MCC (Millennium Challenge Corporation). 2010. *About the MCC.* http://www.mcc.gov/pages/about (accessed September 23, 2010).

McNeil, D. 2010. At front lines, AIDS war is falling apart. *The New York Times.*

Nye, J. S. 2006 (unpublished). *Soft power, hard power and leadership.* Harvard University.

Office of the Global AIDS Coordinator. 2008. *Guidance for PEPFAR partnership frameworks and partnership framework implementation plans (version 2.0).* Washington, DC: PEPFAR.

———. 2009. *The U.S. President's Emergency Plan for AIDS Relief: Five-year strategy.* Washington, DC: PEPFAR.

Oomman, N., M. Bernstein, and S. Rosenzweig. 2007. *Following the funding for HIV/AIDS: A comparative analysis of the funding practices of PEPFAR, the Global Fund and World Bank MAP in Mozambique, Uganda and Zambia.* Washington, DC: Center for Global Development.

Over, M. 2008. *Prevention failure: The ballooning entitlement burden of U.S. global AIDS treatment spending and what to do about it.* Washington, DC: Center for Global Development.

PEPFAR (U.S. President's Emergency Plan for AIDS Relief). 2009a. *Celebrating life: Fifth annual report to Congress on PEPFAR (2009).* Washington, DC: PEPFAR.

———. 2009b. *World AIDS day 2009: Latest PEPFAR results (December 2009).* Washington, DC: PEPFAR.

———. 2010. *Sixth annual report to Congress on PEPFAR program results.* Washington, DC: PEPFAR.

Pew Research Center. 2008. *Global public opinion in the Bush years (2001-2008).* Washington, DC: Pew Research Center.

Ray, J. 2008. *U.S. Leadership approval highest in sub-Saharan Africa.* Gallup. http://www.gallup.com/poll/106306/us-leadership-approval-highest-subsaharan-africa.aspx (accessed June 8, 2010).

SABCOHA (South African Business Coalition on HIV/AIDS). 2010. *Who we are.* http://www.sabcoha.org/who-we-are/who-we-are.html (accessed September 24, 2010).

Stolberg, S. G. 2008. In global battle on AIDS, Bush creates a legacy. *The New York Times.*

Summers, T. 2002. *The Global Fund to fight AIDS, TB, and malaria: Challenges and opportunities.* Washington, DC: CSIS.

The White House. 2010. *National security strategy.* Washington, DC: The White House. http://www.whitehouse.gov/sites/default/files/rss_viewer/national_security_strategy.pdf (accessed July 12, 2010).

Tutu, D. 2010. Obama's overdue AIDS bill. *The New York Times.*

UNAIDS (The Joint United Nations Programme on HIV/AIDS). 2010. *Global report: UNAIDS report on the global AIDS epidemic 2010.* Geneva: UNAIDS.

UNAIDS and WHO (The Joint United Nations Programme on HIV/AIDS and World Health Organization). 2009. *AIDS epidemic update: December 2009.* Geneva: UNAIDS.

UNGASS (United Nations General Assembly Special Session). 2001. Declaration of commitment on HIV/AIDS, 27 June 2001. http://data.unaids.org/publications/irc-pub03/aidsdeclaration_en.pdf (accessed September 7, 2010).

UNITAID. 2010. *UNITAID approves patent pool.* http://www.unitaid.eu/en/20091215237/News/UNITAID-APPROVES-PATENT-POOL.html (accessed October 19, 2010).

USAID (United States Agency for International Development). 2009a. *Kenya fact sheet: FY 2008-11 USAID-state foreign assistance appropriations.* Washington, DC: USAID.

———. 2009b. *Nigeria fact sheet: FY 2008-11 USAID-state foreign assistance appropriations.* Washington, DC: USAID.

———. 2009c. *Rwanda fact sheet: FY 2008-11 USAID-state foreign assistance appropriations.* Washington, DC: USAID.

———. 2009d. *Uganda fact sheet: FY 2008-11 USAID-state foreign assistance appropriations.* Washington, DC: USAID.

Voice of America. 2010. *Obama criticized over AIDS funding.* National Public Radio.

Ward, J. 2007. Bush to visit Africa to see fruit of U.S. AIDS funding. *The Washington Times*, December 1.

Whiteside, A., and A. Whalley. 2007. *Reviewing "emergencies" for Swaziland: Shifting the paradigm in a new era.* Mbabane and Durban: National Emergency Response Council on HIV/AIDS (NERCHA) and Health Economics & HIV/AIDS Research Division (HEARD).

WHO, UNAIDS, and UNICEF. 2009. *Towards universal access: Scaling up priority HIV/AIDS interventions in the health sector, progress report 2009.* Geneva: WHO.

World Bank. 2008. *World development report: Agriculture for development.* Washington, DC: World Bank.

Zakumumpa, H. 2010. Thousands risk early death as AIDS care centres turn away new patients. *The Independent.*

4

The Burden of HIV/AIDS: Implications for African States and Societies

Key Findings

- The burden of HIV/AIDS has profound implications for four sectors of African society: development, health, the state, and academia.
- These impacts confronting many African states and societies pose challenges to their management of their epidemics now and into the future.
- The mosaic of African nations is significantly heterogeneous in the extent of the HIV/AIDS burden and its implications.

In 2009, an estimated 1.8 million new HIV infections occurred in Africa (UNAIDS, 2010), accounting for 69 percent of new infections worldwide; in the same year, 370,000 children began their lives with HIV, which is a decrease from the previous year when 390,000 African children were infected through mother-to-child transmission (UNAIDS, 2010; UNAIDS and WHO, 2009). Between December 2008 and December 2009, 961,000 patients in Africa began receiving antiretroviral therapy (ART), bringing the total receiving treatment to 3,911,000, just 36 percent of those in need of treatment in Africa according to the 2010 guidelines of the World Health Organization (WHO) (WHO et al., 2010). In 2009, 1.3 million Africans lost their lives as a result of AIDS[1] (UNAIDS, 2010). Also in

---

[1] This number could be an underestimation as official death certificates often do not cite AIDS as the cause of death.

Care Options for Orphans and Vulnerable Children

Although recent data are scarce as to who is caring for orphaned African children, it appears that throughout Africa, household-based care is dominant (Subbarao and Coury, 2004). Most orphans reside in foster care within family lines. Foster care and adoption by nonrelatives are uncommon, in part because of a variety of cultural beliefs and taboos. Institutional care for orphans also is quite limited, although it appears to be growing in some countries. According to a recent Save the Children report from Liberia, there are 11 times more orphanages now than 20 years ago. In Zimbabwe, 24 new care institutions for children were built between 1994 and 2004, and the number of children in residential care doubled. In Ghana, the number of such homes increased from 10 in 1996 to more than 140 in 2009 (Csáky, 2009).

One reason for the relatively limited number of institutionalized care facilities for orphans is the cost of running them. The cost per child per year ranges from US $5,403 (with donated food) in Rwanda to $1,350 in Eritrea and $698 in Burundi. Placing just 1 percent of the 508,000 Burundian orphans in such institutions would cost $3.5 million each year. For most African countries, this cost per child rules out institutions as the preferred option for scaling up of orphan care (Csáky, 2009). A 2001 study comparing the cost-effectiveness of six models of orphan care in South Africa found that formal institutional care is the least cost-effective model, while informal models, such as community-based care and informal fostering, are relatively more cost-effective, although they fail to meet minimum standards of care (Desmond and Gow, 2001). Other studies have reached similar conclusions (Owiti, 2004; Subbarao and Coury, 2004).

Given the diverse cultural and socioeconomic settings in Africa and the complex needs of orphans and vulnerable children, most countries are adopting a cost-effective care model that considers multiple levels of care. In Malawi, for example, the National Orphans Task Force has developed a guideline for orphan care in which community-based programs are at the forefront of interventions, followed by foster care; institutional care is the last-resort option, as a temporary measure (Subbarao and Coury, 2004).

Policy Implications with a Long-Term Perspective

According to Booysen (2004a), dedicated resources that target HIV/AIDS-affected households with broad-based medical, educational, and social security systems could potentially prevent these households from declining into chronic poverty. The stakes of such policies are potentially very high for African countries' long-term economic development. Bell and colleagues (2004) contend that "AIDS does much more . . . than destroy the existing abilities and capacities—the human capital—embodied in its victims; it also weakens the mechanism in which human capital is formed in the next generation and beyond." Children deprived of adequate childrearing and education will transfer their capacity and knowledge gaps to their own children, thereby transmitting and amplifying the HIV/AIDS-generated poverty trap in generations to come. Using projections from two high-prevalence countries, Bell and colleagues conclude that without aggressive and expensive policies to preserve the development and transfer of human capital in overlapping generations, highly affected countries risk progressive collapse of their economies. A recent review of studies in Tanzania and Uganda (Seeley et al., 2010) confirms lasting negative impacts on household poverty and on children, but does not confirm large societal impacts of the order predicted by Bell and colleagues (2004). Nevertheless, the latter authors' focus on the injurious effects of HIV/AIDS from generation to generation rightly underscores the epidemic's significance for Africa's future.

Economic Performance

HIV is sexually transmitted, debilitating, and fatal. Most of the sickness and death caused by the infection is in adults of (re)productive age. Even scholars who doubt the pertinence of disease for economic growth concede that these facts about HIV/AIDS compel special consideration in macroeconomic analyses for countries with generalized and severe epidemics (Acemoglu and Johnson, 2007). Alongside orphaning with its lasting effects, HIV/AIDS-related adult morbidity and premature death affect economic development in several direct and indirect ways.

Labor and Productivity

The disease's impacts on labor and productivity are immediately relevant. In a study of HIV/AIDS and private-sector companies in Africa, Feeley and colleagues (2009) describe a variety of costs to businesses. Employee absenteeism and impaired function due to HIV/AIDS represent tangible costs to companies operating in highly affected communities. Both lead to lower productivity, the cost of which is felt most strongly by firms relying on skilled labor and having invested in worker training. Other costs to companies take the form of increased employee benefits (whether for treatment or for benefits to families in the event of death), costs of recruiting new staff, and increased management time spent on HIV/AIDS-related issues of infected employees. In the pre-ART era, empirical reviews of these extra costs to companies—the "AIDS tax"—showed them to account for 0.5 to 10.8 percent of total compensation costs, depending on the HIV/AIDS burden in the community and the workforce (Feeley et al., 2009). Although a 1–2 percent "AIDS tax" is more common, companies aware of these costs often seek ways to mitigate, cut, or shift these extra expenses (Barks-Ruggles et al., 2001; Reddy and Swanepoel, 2006; Rosen et al., 2007).

Following the initiation of ART, some loss of productivity may result from the treatment itself, whether because of toxicities (side effects) of the antiretro-viral (ARV) drugs or the queuing time required to obtain services in the public sector (queues at public clinics can last for many hours, and current ART guide-lines typically require many clinic visits, especially in the first year) (Rosen et al., 2007). On the other hand, some data suggest that—using worker absenteeism as a proxy for productivity—ART is effective in restoring the productivity of infected workers over time (Habyarimana et al., 2010; Rosen et al., 2010).

Within the private sector, reduced labor performance combined with increased labor costs may discourage business investment in communities with severe epidemics (Arbache, 2009). A vicious cycle may ensue, whereby the disease negatively impacts labor supply and performance, leading to negative impacts on capital investment, leading to a decline in employment. As household incomes decline, a high burden of HIV/AIDS can ultimately lead to negative market impacts (Feeley et al., 2009).

Economic Growth

While the economic impact of HIV/AIDS on households is well established, so is their remarkable ability to cope. Although potentially consequential for an individual entrepreneur, high morbidity and mortality among the labor force do not necessarily slow the overall macroeconomic growth of an economy as long as new firms arise to replace those hurt by the epidemic, and new healthy, equally productive employees are hired to replace those lost to illness and death. Many African economies suffer from extreme unemployment and underemploy-ment of their labor forces, so firms may be able to replace lost workers at a low cost. Given that enterprise surveys in Africa typically find turnover rates among unskilled workers of around 11 percent per year in the absence of HIV/AIDS, a very high HIV prevalence is required to substantially increase annual hiring costs. Thus, the question of whether a high prevalence of HIV infection reduces per capita economic growth remains pertinent.

Early analyses of the economic impact of the HIV/AIDS epidemic down-played its consequences for GDP (Lovász and Schipp, 2009). Researchers drew these conclusions largely because of the way they assessed GDP (per capita GDP = GDP/total population), which takes into account the size of the popula-tion. With this formula, when the growth rate of the population declined along with GDP, a minimal economic impact of HIV/AIDS was found. Many of these studies were conducted at a time when the morbidity and mortality from HIV had not been fully realized. Newer analysis approaches take into account more recent data and use advanced modeling techniques. Using these approaches, several authors have found statistically significant negative effects of HIV prevalence on the growth of per capita GDP. One of the most methodologically sophisticated of these efforts is a recent study by McDonald and Roberts (2006), who found the negative effects of HIV/AIDS on economic growth in Africa to be statistically significant. In their model, using data from the pretreatment era, poor health and loss of life reduce social and economic capital. In the Africa sample, an average reduction of 0.59 percent in income per capita results from a 1 percent increase in HIV prevalence (McDonald and Roberts, 2006). In contrast to reports reviewed by Feeley and colleagues (2009), the findings of McDonald and Roberts show that surplus labor supplies in poor countries do not diminish the negative effects of HIV/AIDS on economic growth. Slower growth reduces the tax base, while every new HIV/AIDS-related illness episode, death, and vulnerable child has financial implications for the public health and social sectors (Arbache, 2009; Haacker, 2006).

Lovász and Schipp (2009) also found a significant negative effect of the HIV/AIDS epidemic on the growth rate of per capita GDP in Africa. Their study—looking at the impact of the epidemic on the pace of economic growth in 41 countries—reports that the economic impact of HIV is not uniform across countries or even within countries. The economies of countries with low HIV prevalence appear able to absorb the shock of the epidemic and maintain relatively normal economic relationships. By contrast, the economies of countries with high prevalence, particularly in southern Africa, experience severe and significant difficulties due to the epidemic (Lovász and Schipp, 2009).

A crucial point that should not be lost in technical discussions of per capita GDP is that HIV/AIDS has a disastrous impact on the social and economic well-being of heavily impacted nations and on their development. The epidemic is reducing the stock of skills, experience, and human capital and, in turn, driving up costs and decreasing productivity (Nkomo, 2010). It is diverting resources away from savings and investment, interrupting generational transfers of knowledge, weakening the education system, and threatening food and human security. All these factors have a long-lasting effect on social and economic development and make it difficult for southern Africa to attain the Millennium Development Goals of eradicating poverty and achieving sustainable development.

Influence of Treatment on Household and Economic Well-Being

Whether for assessing ART's effect on preventing orphanhood and vulnerability in children or on averting affronts to African economies, understanding the influence of treatment on the socioeconomic impacts of HIV/AIDS has now become imperative. One of the first studies of this kind examines the impact of treatment on labor supply in a rural region of western Kenya (Thirumurthy et al., 2008). Within 6 months of treatment initiation, adult labor supply and participation among HIV/AIDS patients increased dramatically. Simultaneously, labor participation of children in the patient's household, especially that of boys, decreased significantly. The effects of the latter finding are larger and impact more household members in households with multiple patients (Thirumurthy et al., 2008).

A review of studies of the economic and quality-of-life outcomes of HIV/ AIDS treatment in developing countries reports similar trends (Beard et al., 2009). Such studies consistently show improvements in physical health after treatment, as well as improvements in subjective well-being and outcomes related to depression, dementia, and anxiety. Other benefits reported in studies reviewed by Beard and colleagues include significant declines in absenteeism after 1 year of ART, coupled with increased work performance. These effects are found across different sectors. Other household-level benefits are reported as well. With increased ability to work among HIV-infected adults, child labor participation declined and school attendance increased. The first 6 months of treatment was also associated with increased consumption of nutritious foods in the household and with a decline in wasting among children under age 5—from 12 percent at baseline to 5 percent after the adult caretaker had been on ART for 5 months.

In South Africa, Booysen (2004b) investigated the role of social grants in mitigating the socioeconomic impact of HIV/AIDS at the household level (Booysen, 2004b). He concluded that social grants play an important role in alleviating poverty (bringing very poor people closer to the poverty line) in HIV-affected households, more so than in eradicating poverty (lifting people out of poverty). However, Booysen notes that the magnitude of the epidemic in South Africa also necessitates consideration of the fiscal affordability and sustainability of such a system in the longer term.

IMPLICATIONS FOR THE HEALTH SECTOR

The concept of the burden of HIV/AIDS is more meaningful if grounded in concrete consequences and resource demands (Parikh and Veenstra, 2008). Nowhere are the consequences of HIV/AIDS and the resulting resource implications more evident than in the health sector. The health sector has long been key in the response to HIV/AIDS, but its role has become more central with the relatively recent addition of clinic-based prevention, treatment, and care services.

Provision of treatment and care is pivotal to managing generalized and severe HIV/AIDS epidemics, and for many African countries, funding commitments for WHO's 3 by 5 Initiative in 2003 represent a turning point in this regard. Financial resources in and of themselves do not make for success, however. Management and institutional capacity demands on the health sector are both substantial and evolving within a changing context of more treatment and care. The injection of resources for HIV/AIDS care, while providing tremendous opportunity to respond more effectively to the epidemic, also presents critical dilemmas concerning the sustainability of service provision over time and the future direction of HIV/AIDS policies and programs. This section reviews some of the challenges and possible trade-offs faced by the health sector in African countries in planning and managing responses to the epidemic.

Supply and Demand, Costs and Benefits

Changes in the supply and demand of health care are one macro-level expression of a shifting HIV/AIDS burden. Early in the global scale-up of treatment and care, Over (2004) described how HIV-related disease both increases demand for and reduces the supply of health sector outputs. The result is health care scarcity, leading to higher costs and national spending for health. Dedicated funding to increase access to HIV/AIDS treatment and care introduces another dynamic. As the supply of HIV/AIDS-related treatment and care increases, so, too, does demand for the new services. While increased supply and demand of HIV/AIDS treatment and care are partially offset by declining demand for treatment of opportunistic infections, they also can cause declines in supply in other health areas (Over, 2004). The provision of complex lifelong treatment to an ever-expanding number of patients will only continue to create extra demand for health care resources, driving up provider incomes and the price of all health care.

On the other hand, evidence from Brazil, where an early response to HIV/AIDS included universal access to ART for medically eligible patients, suggests that aggressively "fighting HIV/AIDS is good business" (Teixeira et al., 2004). As has been seen in wealthier contexts (Gebo et al., 2005; Krentz et al., 2006; Sherer et al., 2002), putting more HIV-infected people on ART in Brazil dramatically reduced deaths and HIV/AIDS-related hospital admissions (Candiani et al., 2007; Teixeira et al., 2004), saving the country's public health sector close to $2 billion between 1997 and 2003 (Teixeira et al., 2004). Reductions in opportunistic infections also were seen with the introduction of ART, suggesting similar potential benefits in African settings (Badri et al., 2002; Jerene et al., 2006). Some scholars question the applicability of Brazil's experience with cost savings for those African countries most challenged by HIV/AIDS (Over, 2004), while others argue that treating more people sooner results in net savings regardless of setting (Ford et al., 2009). Empirical evidence for both arguments is lacking, however.

While the cost/benefit debate continues, there is no question as to the clinical benefits of earlier treatment, as reflected in WHO's recent recommendation to initiate ART earlier at a CD4 threshold of 350 cells/μL for all HIV-positive patients regardless of symptoms (WHO, 2009). In addition to the clinical benefits for individual patients, many experts believe that treating more people earlier also has a prevention benefit (see the discussion below and in Chapter 2), although this benefit is still under debate (Cohen and Gay, 2010; Mastro and Cohen, 2010; World Bank and USAID, 2010). Moreover, treating key coinfections decreases viral load, which has been shown to slow HIV progression; even small changes in viral load could translate into population-level benefits in lowering the risk of HIV transmission (Lingappa et al., 2010; Modjarrad and Vermund, 2010).

Strains on the Health System

However compelling the argument for a double—clinical and preventive—or even a triple—clinical, preventive, and cost savings—benefit of ART may be, there is no doubt that the ever-growing number of patients on lifelong treatment is placing significant strains on health systems (Boulle and Ford, 2007), strains that will increasingly be felt by outpatient services at the primary care level (Parikh and Veenstra, 2008). The result could be to detract attention from other essential primary health care services (Van Damme et al., 2006). Even in small countries where ART programs are faring well, the massive commodity, laboratory, and clinic demands associated with chronic disease management for an expanding HIV/AIDS patient population will present daunting challenges in the years ahead (Harries et al., 2006). Regardless of the programmatic successes seen to date, moreover, Veenstra and colleagues (2010) remind us that, in addition to weaknesses in health and drug supply systems, other crises in African countries can further compromise the delivery of ART programs, leading to drug resistance, treatment failure, and additional burdens on the health system. In addition, questions have been raised about whether poor integration of donor support to combat a single disease could weaken host country health systems (Oomman et al., 2008) .

Thus, expanded access to HIV/AIDS treatment and care is in some ways transforming and in other ways amplifying the challenge for African countries. Unfortunately, the infrastructure in most African countries is not based on a chronic care model. The closest example in these countries may be a well-child or tuberculosis clinic (de-Graft Aikins et al., 2010). Effective long-term treatment of HIV/AIDS requires high-functioning health systems equipped with capacities for prolonged laboratory monitoring and integrated patient management to enable regular follow-up and changes in treatment. The service delivery models and expectations of care established decades ago have proven woefully inadequate for responding to the quality and complexity of care demanded for HIV/AIDS (Coovadia and Bland, 2008).

An additional stress on health care systems in Africa is worker migration. The mobility of health care personnel—within countries (from rural to urban locations), between countries (from weaker to stronger economies), to donor organizations and nongovernmental organizations (NGOs) (away from public clinics), and globally (to high-income countries)—further stresses already weak and fragile systems (Awases et al., 2004; Hagopian et al., 2004).

The outcomes of the world's unprecedented effort to address a devastating health issue remain unknown. Over's (2004) predictions of mounting health care demand and intensified health system stressors are well placed, however, and at this juncture demand serious consideration. For African countries whose HIV/AIDS treatment and care programs are largely or wholly dependent on donor aid, a pressing concern now is how to manage the transition in the face of stagnating or decreasing donor assistance. For those rare countries that are shouldering a prominent portion of their health sector's care and treatment burden, the question is how to sustain the response with an unending increase in the number of HIV/AIDS patients needing care. Managing the epidemic effectively will require that political and health leaders confront these questions forthrightly, a process that must begin with grasping the dynamic resource demands for sustaining an adequate response.

Testing Capacity

The significant challenges of sustaining a health sector response to the HIV/AIDS burden begin with testing. Considered the gateway for HIV prevention, treatment, and care, HIV testing has provided a foundation for African countries' management of their epidemics. A negative test result presents an opportunity for primary prevention through test-linked counseling and education; a positive result presents an opportunity for secondary prevention and referral to support, treatment, and care services for patients and affected families.

Recognizing this important opportunity, WHO recommends provider-initiated HIV testing and counseling as part of the routine delivery of primary health care in countries with generalized epidemics (WHO and UNAIDS, 2007). Working toward implementation of this guidance, African countries substantially increased the number of testing centers and the number of tests per 1,000 population between 2007 and 2008 (WHO et al., 2009). While innovative community-, workplace-, and home-based testing approaches have been tried (see Box 4-1), expanded access to HIV testing has required massive investments in health

---

BOX 4-1
Innovative Testing Approaches

An innovative strategy for prevention being used in the Democratic Republic of the Congo is mobile HIV testing. A van—furnished with a sampling chair, a refrigerator, a laboratory, and a generator—arrives in public places such as markets and major intersections for immediate and free testing. The van is often surrounded by curious onlookers, and this basic system has encouraged many people to learn their HIV status. Those who test positive are referred to care centers (Séverin, 2010). Similarly, in Benin, The World Bank supports two mobile laboratories, equipped with a spectrophotometer and a cyflow, to help meet the increasing demand for HIV screening. The mobile laboratories facilitate the collection of blood samples in the most remote areas of the country and transport the samples to laboratories for screening (Afrique Avenir, 2010).

system infrastructure (private consultation rooms and upgraded laboratories), more health personnel (counselors and laboratory technicians), improved supply chain systems (to move reagents, test kits, and medical supplies), additional record-keeping functions, and improved referral systems. Yet despite the investments made to date and improved capacities to perform HIV testing, access to testing remains considerably below desired levels. Moreover, the test is merely a starting point for more complex and costly interventions. Benefit does not accrue from testing alone, but from successful referral to treatment and care of those found to be HIV-positive. While clearly essential to managing and controlling African epidemics, broader access to HIV testing has altered the resource demand landscape and presented critical new challenges for African health leaders to consider.

Need for Mental Health Care

Mental health conditions have been described as both a risk factor for and a consequence of HIV (Bodibe, 2010; Meade and Sikkema, 2005). Among patients with HIV infection, depression is the most frequently observed psychiatric disorder (Nakasujja et al., 2010). Cognitive impairment in HIV patients also is common, ranging from minor cognitive motor disorder to HIV dementia. Studies conducted in Africa have found alarmingly high rates of dementia in HIV-positive patients (Freeman et al., 2007; Wong et al., 2007). This finding raises great concern not only because the condition is treatable if recognized, but also because HIV-associated dementia can have adverse effects on adherence to HIV treatment.

Given the projected large numbers of people who will be diagnosed and living with HIV/AIDS in the next decade, the need for a strong mental health and neurological workforce is evident. According to the joint IOM/Uganda National Academy of Sciences workshop summary *Mental, Neurological, and Substance Use Disorders in Sub-Saharan Africa: Reducing the Treatment Gap, Improving Quality of Care* (IOM, 2010), the low-income countries of Africa have very few of these skilled professionals available to treat the large numbers of persons with such disorders. The report emphasizes the paucity of trained professionals in this field compared with developed nations:

> In the clinical neurosciences (neurologists, neurosurgeons, psychiatrists), except for South Africa, the mean ratios for countries that have these medical specialists are 1 neurologist for 1 million to 2.8 million people (versus 4 per 100,000 in Europe); 1 psychiatrist for 900,000 people (versus 9 per 100,000 in Europe); and 1 neurosurgeon for 2 million to 6 million people (versus 1 per 100,000 in Europe). Most of the clinical neuroscience services are located in the capital cities, often the largest urban areas, where the professionals also often lecture at the medical schools. As a result MNS patients often must travel long distances to consult with a doctor in the city (IOM, 2010; Silberberg and Katabira, 2006).

Need for Social Services

Given the number of highly vulnerable children in Africa and the limited capacity of its child welfare sector, some have suggested that investments are needed to build a cadre of professionals and paraprofessionals with social work skills (Khumalo, 2009; Lombard, 2008; USAID, 2009). Yet few particulars are known about the child welfare sector and the social work workforce in Africa, and there have been few country projections of the demand for these services and related workforce needs.

The Global Health Bureau of the U.S. Agency for International Development (USAID) commissioned a study to assess the opportunities for and constraints on building the social work workforce within the child welfare sector in Africa (USAID, 2009). A key observation resulting from this study is the existence of a historically rich social work profession in Africa built on a community ideology and focused on meeting the needs of vulnerable children and families, especially those living in poverty. At the same time, the study identified the underdevelopment of the profession and the need to build the capacity of child welfare and social work education systems in Africa.

As with the profession in general, little is known about social work education in Africa. The available data are anecdotal and self-reported, and obtaining accurate and current information on the numbers of schools, students, and graduates is difficult. However, the projected shortfalls of graduates suggest the need for systematic evaluation of the capacity of African social work education (USAID, 2009). Evaluation of social work teaching methods and curricula also appears to be needed. Several apparent shortcomings have been noted: many faculty received training in the West and are therefore more familiar with the Western literature than their own indigenous knowledge; social work teaching methods tend to lack the participatory models necessary to engage students in active problem solving; and field education experiences in rural community settings are inadequate (Hochfeld et al., 2009; USAID, 2009).

Health Systems: Needs and Opportunities

WHO's *Global Strategy for Health for All by the Year 2000* called for strengthening health systems through sound coordination mechanisms combined with adequate infrastructure, human resources, logistics support, and referral and health information systems (WHO, 1981). Thirty years after this call to action, weaknesses in African health systems have been identified as the major obstacle to reaching WHO's 3 by 5 treatment targets (Schneider et al., 2006; Van Damme et al., 2006).

Not only are weak health systems a baseline problem, but they are also at risk of undergoing further weakening and distortion from HIV/AIDS-focused interventions (De Maeseneer et al., 2008; McCoy et al., 2005). Recent concern about the potential of HIV/AIDS programs to undermine public health systems is part of a long-standing debate over disease-specific versus health system approaches (Freedman, 2005; Unger et al., 2003; Van Balen, 2004). Yet while some negative effects on health coordination and harmonization have been reported with the implementation of HIV/AIDS treatment and care initiatives (Biesma et al., 2009), a growing evidence base shows mainly positive contributions of these initiatives to key functions of health systems (Embrey et al., 2009; Harries et al., 2009; Sherr et al., 2009; Yu et al., 2008).

Specifically, Embrey and colleagues (2009) describe how the great need for HIV/AIDS-related products for treatment and care scale-up in Africa has led to improved capacities in pharmaceutical procurement and supply chain systems more generally, although a number of interrelated constraints in procurement and supply management remain. In particular, recurrent "stockouts" of ARV drugs are common among almost all health facilities in west and central Africa, mainly as a result of inadequate forecasting and information flow among stakeholders (UNICEF et al., 2008). A similar situation has been noted in east and southern Africa, where stockouts of ARVs and other life-saving drugs have also been a problem (IRIN, 2010; Thom and Langa, 2010).

HIV/AIDS care similarly demands improved laboratory capacities at all levels of the health care system (Spira et al., 2009), as well as better medical record keeping and data management (Forster et al., 2008). Supply chains, laboratories, and medical records are basic components of any health care system. For many African countries, new attention to these essential system components represents catching up to basic standards as much as meeting special demands for managing HIV/AIDS patients. Moreover, while more evidence is needed on the impact of HIV/AIDS programs on service delivery in other health areas, data from Rwanda (Price et al., 2009) and Haiti (Walton et al., 2004) suggest an association between the introduction of HIV/AIDS care and increased delivery and uptake of other primary health care services. Conversely, a recent retrospective analysis of publicly available WHO data found little or no country-level impact of PEPFAR funding on non-HIV/AIDS health outcomes that were not explicitly targeted (Duber et al., 2010).

While both positive and negative effects of AIDS funding have been asserted, available evidence on the effects of the scaled-up response to HIV/AIDS on health systems is slim. Many arguments suggesting impacts of HIV investments on health systems are based on anecdotes and speculation, on small pilots, or on early stages of programs that cannot yet be generalized, and a number of systematic impact studies are still under way (Yu et al., 2008). Therefore, the question of positive, negative, or neutral spillover effects of HIV/AIDS-targeted programs remains an important topic that demands further examination (Rabkin et al., 2009). At the same time, Jeena (2005) and Bodkin and colleagues (2006) remind us that in and of itself, HIV/AIDS care is an important aspect of maternal and child health care.

Human resource demands related to HIV/AIDS care remain a significant concern. (See Chapter 5 for further discussion of the human resource crisis in Africa.) In Africa, HIV/AIDS adds to the demand for and sometimes decreases the supply of health workers (Herbst et al., 2009). For example, HIV in health workers is a contributing factor to absenteeism, resulting not just from the primary HIV infection but also from immunocompromised workers' increased risk of occupationally acquired illnesses such as tuberculosis (including its multi- and extensively drug-resistant forms). Poor infection control practices leading to these infections place further strains on the health care system. From a resource perspective, a key element of health system strengthening is protection of the health care workforce—in the same way that any scarce resource would be protected.

Although multiple actions are needed to address systemic problems of production, retention, and allocation of health workers (Philips et al., 2008), scaling up of HIV/AIDS treatment and care has resulted in several innovations in care delivery in Africa. Substantial evidence shows that alternatives to physician-centered treatment, such as community-based support for patient enrollment and follow-up (Sanjana et al., 2009; Torpey et al., 2008), are both feasible and effective (Bedula et al., 2007; Gimbel-Sherr et al., 2007; Sanne et al., 2010; Shumbusho et al., 2009; Stringer et al., 2006). Tasks related to initiating and managing ART often are shifted to nurses, with good clinical outcomes, and there is some evidence that other nonphysicians, such as clinical officers (who have 3 years of clinical and practical training beyond grade 12) can also fill this need (Bolton-Moore et al., 2007).

Researchers in Uganda estimated the cost and personnel impact of task shifting from physicians to nurses and pharmacy workers for ART follow-up. They demonstrated a US $0.5–11.0 million savings and the freeing up of 4.1–14.8 percent of nationally available physician full-time equivalents (FTEs) annually. Applying the same methodology to all of Africa—with 9.7 million patients in need of ART (31 percent access) and 150,714 practicing physicians—the researchers found that task shifting could save $0.476–2.769 billion and free up 4.1–5.9 percent of available physician FTEs on the continent (Harling et al., 2007).

Overall, documentation of positive effects of HIV/AIDS programs on African health systems suggests that recent investments in treatment and care are beginning to fill unmet system needs dating back to WHO's strategic plan to operationalize the declaration of Alma Ata. While aid recipients and donors alike need to overcome weaknesses in coordination and health governance with respect to HIV/AIDS (Spicer et al., 2010), the benefits to health systems might be expected to amplify over time as programs mature and services become mainstreamed.

Prevention: A Necessary Health Sector Priority

Attention needs to be focused not on the false debate pitting health systems against disease-specific interventions and primary health care against HIV/AIDS care, but on the overarching question of how many more new HIV/AIDS patients even the best-resourced and best-performing health systems can absorb and provide with quality care. The essential problem for African countries is unchecked HIV incidence. HIV infection and associated diseases are overwhelming health systems, and there is an urgent need to curb new transmissions. Now more than ever, strong health systems with sophisticated patient management capacities are needed in Africa not only to care for HIV-infected patients, but also to deliver biomedical and behavioral prevention services.

As discussed in Chapter 2, whether to focus resources on prevention or treatment is another false debate (Creese et al., 2002; Marseille et al., 2002). The ability of countries to sustain treatment programs will require averting more new infections, and ART as pre- and postexposure prophylaxis rather than just for therapeutic purposes will be critical in holistic prevention strategies. A comprehensive response that balances prevention, treatment, support, and care is needed. This response must include a strong emphasis on the disclosure of prevention outcomes. African nations need to share their prevention experiences and best practices with one another; greater transparency on the part of African ministries of health in disclosing their countries' prevention outcomes and impacts would help create a demand for prevention.

Nearly two decades ago, Cates and Hinman (1992) advocated for all-inclusive prevention strategies drawing on the full range of technologies and approaches available at the time. Leaders in the field continue to make the same plea for approaches that link prevention, treatment, and care (Piot et al., 2008). Prevention is in everyone's interest, including HIV-infected persons. Predicting the difficult questions and trade-offs now confronting African countries with severe epidemics and high treatment burdens, Over (2004) suggests that "to the extent that HIV-positive groups assist in reducing new infections, they will help ensure the affordability of continued treatment and thus serve their own long-term interests."

IMPLICATIONS FOR THE STATE

A product of the world's most recent, efficient, in many ways brutal, and short-lived colonial encounters, modern African states have long faced challenges to their security, capacity, and attempts at democracy (Young, 1994). The severity of HIV/AIDS epidemics in many African countries and the disease's potential to have long-term negative societal effects have exacerbated these challenges and have provoked multidisciplinary investigation of the consequences of HIV for African states (de Waal, 2010; Patterson, 2005a). While the gravest predictions of national vulnerabilities stemming from high infection rates and HIV/AIDS-related deaths have largely been revised, the implications of the epidemic for state security and governance in Africa remain pertinent and in some countries possibly profound.

Security and Conflict

As the scale of HIV/AIDS epidemics became apparent, concerns about how the disease influences armed conflict and security increased. Presumed high infection rates in the armed forces produced concerns that national militaries would be weakened by HIV/AIDS-related deaths, that infected troops were a source of infection of the general population, and that war and conflict were associated with the spread of the disease (Eboko, 2005; Whiteside et al., 2006). The evidence supporting these concerns, however, is inconsistent.

One review of data from 21 African countries found that in all cases, the prevalence of HIV/AIDS was similar or higher in military samples compared with the general population, and in some countries dramatically so (Ba et al., 2008). Recruits in all the samples further showed higher prevalence compared with the general population of males aged 15–24. These findings contradict an analysis published 2 years previously by Whiteside and colleagues (2006), which challenges the common wisdom as to the impact of HIV/AIDS on the security of African states. Referring to available data on HIV infection in the military as of 2006, the authors argue that new recruits and serving soldiers have infection rates paralleling those of their civilian counterparts. In a recent report on studies commissioned by the AIDS, Security and Conflict Initiative, de Waal (2010) also questions findings and assumptions that the prevalence of HIV/AIDS is higher among armed forces than in civilian populations and concludes that fears of much-elevated HIV rates among soldiers, with disastrous impacts on armies as institutions, have been overstated. For example, regarding the assumption that high losses of troops to HIV/AIDS were endangering the functioning of national armies, the authors contend that the "built-in redundancy" in armies, which expect casualties in times of war, protects military forces from weakening because of disease-related deaths, as do policies to discharge HIV-positive soldiers (Whiteside et al., 2006).

The assumption that war and conflict contribute to the spread of HIV has also been questioned. A study commissioned by the AIDS, Security and Conflict Initiative found no correlation, for example, between conflict and war and national HIV/AIDS prevalence rates (de Waal, 2010). Further, with the exception of the 1994 genocide in Rwanda (Ba et al., 2008), command-approved sexual violence whereby HIV-infected troops are deployed for rape has not been reported in conflict situations (Whiteside et al., 2006). However, studies conducted for the AIDS, Security and Conflict Initiative that focus on the gender impact of conflict suggest that the link between sexual violence and HIV has yet to be fully understood and that gender-associated vulnerabilities remain inadequately conceptualized (de Waal, 2010). Additionally, more attention to postconflict conditions that may favor the spread of HIV/AIDS is needed, including gender-associated vulnerabilities in periods of postconflict transition (de Waal, 2010; Whiteside et al., 2006).

State Capacity and Governance

Like national security concerns, the impact of Africa's HIV/AIDS epidemic on state capacity and governance systems has received attention in the last decade. High numbers of HIV-infected citizens can affect governance in several ways, such as through the loss of civil servants and political representatives, the depletion of social networks, the high cost of treatment programs and dependence on donor aid to finance and sustain such programs, and citizens' discontent with the inability of government to provide services. A limited but growing literature examines such issues.

State Capacity and Citizen Expectations

Early predictions of how HIV/AIDS might negatively affect African governance were often quite dire. According to de Waal (2003), by undermining civil society, fueling intergroup tensions, and straining governance systems through mounting demand for programs, severe epidemics could impede the building of capable states in Africa, possibly halting or reversing "the Weberian model of modernity, progressing from traditional or charismatic authority to rational bureaucratic power" (p. 12). Moreover, de Waal suggested that, instead of bolstering rapidly changing African states, major inflows of new HIV/AIDS-dedicated aid resources would present substantial management burdens that could further compromise state capacities.

As with prior assumptions about the impact of HIV/AIDS on security and conflict in Africa, understanding of the consequences of the epidemic for state capacity and governance has been revised and become more nuanced over time. Overall, HIV/AIDS-induced crises in capacity and governance in highly affected countries have yet to materialize. A main reason for this is that, relative to other pressing social issues, HIV/AIDS simply is not a priority for most African citizens (de Waal, 2007; Patterson, 2006). In 2008, respondents in the Malawi Longitudinal Study of Families and Health—conducted as part of the Afrobarometer survey—were asked to rank the importance of five public policy priorities. AIDS services ranked last among the five. The most important priority was clean water, followed by agricultural development, health services, and education (Dionne et al., 2008). One important exception is HIV/AIDS treatment activism in South Africa (Patterson, 2006). More often, however, competing social and economic needs, combined with continued denial and stigmatization of HIV/AIDS in some countries, have constrained public demand for HIV/AIDS-related services. Furthermore, underdevelopment of democratic institutions has limited citizen demand for state accountability for a response to the epidemic. It is not surprising, then, that case studies in Uganda, Swaziland, South Africa, and Zimbabwe found that elected officials did not fear repercussions in elections as a result of a lack of attention to the epidemic and its consequences (Patterson, 2006).

The most recent studies resulting from the AIDS, Security and Conflict Initiative also discount links between HIV/AIDS and state fragility, capacity, and quality of governance at the national level. The studies do, however, provide evidence that negative impacts are being felt at the subnational and local levels. In a summary of these studies, de Waal (2010) describes situations of increasing pressure on local governments to expand the quantity and scope of HIV/AIDS-related services as "vortices of crisis" that in some contexts are contributing to poor service delivery to the public. He concludes that there is an urgent need to mitigate this impact on local governments and communities and to enhance service delivery in weak and struggling states.

Albeit inadequately documented, most evidence to date suggests a feedback loop of low state responsiveness to the epidemic, which begins with low public demand around the disease and its immediate consequences. That is, minimal public demand for services leads to minimal government commitment. Where an aggressive response is mounted, high dependency on external support is typically necessary. As a result of the combination of citizens' preoccupation with other issues and the international community's support for the response in many African countries, citizen discontent with government's lack of response has yet to be manifested. A reduction or withdrawal of donor aid for recently scaled-up HIV/AIDS care and treatment programs will likely result in fewer services and less patient care; however, the African public's response to losing this new health care entitlement is uncertain (Lyman and Wittels, 2010).

Impacts on Electoral Processes and Outcomes

Although critically important at this juncture of maturing democracies in Africa, empirically based understanding of the impact of HIV/AIDS on electoral processes and outcomes is scarce. Chirambo's (2009) examination of the effects of HIV/AIDS on electoral governance systems in Namibia, Malawi, Senegal, South Africa, Tanzania, and Zambia is an important exception. In studies conducted between 2003 and 2007, Chirambo tested the hypothesis that HIV/AIDS undermines the electoral processes in these countries. Paralleling HIV/AIDS-related deaths in the population in the same age range, the studies presume high mortality among elected representatives (members of parliament [MPs]). While the causes of death among MPs are unknown, Chirambo notes that in the mid-1990s, many southern African countries recorded significant losses of MPs to natural, undisclosed illness.

Chirambo (2009) concludes that HIV/AIDS likely has important consequences for electoral governance, which vary depending on the form of government. Majoritarian systems based on small voting districts require by-elections upon MP losses. As high HIV/AIDS-related mortality accelerates the rate of MP vacancies, majoritarian systems bear the greatest costs in both political and economic terms. Constituencies may lose voice as frequent by-elections attract fewer voters and the organization of multiple by-elections consumes state and political party resources. Having fewer resources to devote to by-elections, smaller parties are especially unable to recapture lost seats and so are disproportionately affected by HIV/AIDS-related deaths relative to larger parties. Governments based on proportional representation, in which large voting areas or an entire country constitutes the constituency, are less burdened by having to hold multiple local by-elections and bear the lowest costs due to HIV/AIDS. Mixed forms of government offer some insulation against high mortality among MPs.

Chirambo's (2009) exploration is unique and important for fully understanding the implications of HIV/AIDS for African states and societies. His analysis of the interaction between HIV/AIDS and political and electoral governance, in particular, provides a starting point for understanding the implications of the epidemic for African countries' transition to democratic forms of government.

Government Responses

Eboko (2005) emphasizes the substantial diversity in African responses to the HIV/AIDS epidemic and cautions against using a generic concept and term— "African"—in describing and understanding those responses. He contends that trends in African epidemics since the early 1980s can essentially be explained by the level of political commitment and proposes the concept of "political culture" to describe the variation in commitment. As the South African state was preoccupied postapartheid by (re)claiming African autonomy, a political culture of "active dissidence" and outright "denial" amounted in effect to low political commitment to mounting an effective HIV/AIDS response. In Côte d'Ivoire and Cameroon, Eboko argues, a political culture of "passive adhesion" resulted in responses led by biomedical professionals that sometimes involved divisions between biomedical elites working with international actors and others working with intended beneficiaries of public health programs. A political culture of "active participation" in Uganda and Senegal represents in many ways the continent's most cohesive and inclusive responses, based on leaders' perceptions of societal networks, both social and scientific.

More than mere theorizing, such intellectual framing of government responses helps us comprehend the variable success in confronting HIV/AIDS in Africa. Given that Uganda had one of the world's most severe epidemics in the 1980s and 1990s, Ugandan state legitimacy and governance could have been compromised. Instead, by embracing an "active participation" response rather than being undermined, the Ugandan state reinforced its legitimacy and governance. Consistent with Eboko's (2005) interpretation, Parkhurst (2005) notes that Uganda reacted early, forcefully, and with a broadly inclusive approach. "By shifting a large portion of its sphere of activity from direct service provision to indirect management, the Ugandan state found an area of policy and intervention that it was able to handle with limited capacity, and which it could undertake without competition from other service providers" (Parkhurst, 2005, p. 583). By assuming the central role of coordinating the inputs of various actors and by not competing with nonstate actors in waging a response, the Ugandan government circumvented challenges to its legitimacy. Repeatedly cited for its good health governance practices, Uganda has also succeeded in mobilizing substantial international financial assistance for HIV/AIDS programs. However, the question of crowding out domestic funding while mobilizing international funding is one that needs to be seriously considered. Some argue that explicit policy choices are behind the crowding out and that the effects unfold very differently depending on the individual countries' situations and choices (Ooms et al., 2010).

A more thorough analysis of African state leadership in the fight against HIV/AIDS lends further clarity to effective state responses. Using Uganda, Swaziland, South Africa, and Zimbabwe as comparative case studies, Patterson (2006) examines leadership on dimensions of centralization of power, neopatrimonialism, state capacity, and security concerns to determine how these elements affect HIV/AIDS policies in those countries. Despite relatively low state stability and capacity, Uganda made a strong HIV/AIDS response effort compared with the other countries. Patterson concludes that the combination of a highly centralized yet inclusive response and high donor funding compensating for low state capacity was key to Uganda's successful response. In particular, President Musevini's early and active engagement in making HIV/AIDS everyone's business helped create a context for broad ownership of and participation in the response.

Complementing Eboko's (2005) analysis, Patterson (2006) explains that despite South Africa's relatively high stability and capacity and decentralized structures, President Mbeki's "state knows best" ideology interfered with an effective early national response to HIV/AIDS. In Swaziland, in contrast with Uganda, high state centralization and neopatrimonialism have compromised the response to the epidemic, as has a mix of "modern" and "traditional" approaches, which are sometimes at odds. Likewise, Zimbabwe's high level of state centralization has had negative effects on the country's HIV/AIDS response. The recent political crisis in the country has displaced HIV-infected persons, interrupting their access to care and treatment services. Power concentrated in the presidency has further curtailed the political space in which HIV/AIDS groups can contribute to policy making and implementation. Given the country's political crisis and high level of neopatrimonialism, the need also has not been filled by external donor support.

Civil Society Participation and Governance Practices

When able to engage in social mobilization, activism, and service delivery, civil society groups can contribute to state capability, accountability, and responsiveness (Jones and Tembo, 2008). However, despite decentralized structures, such as district-level HIV/AIDS committees, and rhetoric in support of community participation and ownership, meaningful civil society participation has often eluded HIV/AIDS programs in Africa.

Civil society's uneven role in the HIV/AIDS response is often linked to weak organizational capacity. In reviewing the characteristics of strong organizations that influence policy, Patterson (2006) cites financial resources, leadership capacity, and internal structures that facilitate transparency and accountability as key. Also important is inclusive networking, capable of creating "united fronts with differing views" and remaining separate from yet collaborating with the state. Possessing all of these characteristics and further bolstered by linkages to global networks, South Africa's Treatment Action Committee is one prominent example of the success of civil society participation in Africa, according to Patterson. Where resources are available and leadership development has been supported, community mobilization can also produce an effective response. Hayes (2009) documents the role of a women's home-based care alliance in Kenya that has focused on partnering with district HIV/AIDS committees to improve the accountability of the HIV/AIDS control program, to secure more resources for home-based care in the community, and to highlight women's contribution to the fight against HIV/AIDS as opposed to their simply being victims of the disease.

An important aspect of programmatic action is the accountability of those in authority. Accountability, however, is too often limited and one-sided, as Harman (2009) illustrates using the World Bank's Multi-Country AIDS Program (MAP). Based on earlier concepts of community development, the MAP was intended to mobilize broad-based community action. Its mandate, however, was to work with states that, in turn, were to enlist community contributions and provide resources for communities to use in taking action through national and local HIV/AIDS committees. Harman's conclusion is that governance of the MAP led to funding delays, top-down decision making with bottom-up and unidirectional accountability (accountability of community groups to the government and the government to the Bank), uneven dialogue and representation of participating organizations, and competition for resources and access to decision making rather than coordination. Such a critical assessment surely cannot be applied across the board to all MAP countries, but it does suggest a need for better understanding of how to engage civil society in an effective multisectoral response to HIV/AIDS.

This example points more generally to a need for broader accountabilities and good health governance practices in responding to HIV/AIDS at the global level (Harman and Lisk, 2009; Patterson, 2005b). In framing a study of the politics of HIV/AIDS in Africa, Patterson (2006) offers the concept of "institutionalizing" the response into a comprehensive political sphere inclusive of the state, civil society (local and global), and bilateral and multilateral donors. That all of these various actors have a long-term interest and political stake in the epidemic is for Patterson the key to institutionalizing the response. Patterson argues that more must be done to institutionalize the fight against HIV/AIDS by addressing questions of unequal power and representation in HIV/AIDS decision making, by empowering civil society associations, and by giving all global citizens a stake in combating the epidemic (Patterson, 2006). Accomplishing this will require not only enduring resource commitments, but also good governance practices. To ensure the most effective use of future resources in the fight against HIV/AIDS, understanding the multiple and variable elements of good governance will be critical for both African countries and donors. More and better documentation of the links between good governance practices and outcomes and impact on the African epidemic is also in order.

IMPLICATIONS FOR ACADEMIA

The need for more trained health care workers to respond to the HIV epidemic is already evident in most African nations and will likely grow as the numbers of people living with HIV/AIDS increase. Obtaining the numbers and types of workers required to meet the unique challenges of each individual country's situation will require planning to determine not only the necessary mix of workers but also the ability of a country's education system—including universities; public health, nursing, and medical schools; technical and vocational institutions; and other academic training programs—to absorb additional students and provide the needed training.

Training for Physicians and Nurses

The need for more physicians and nurses has been well documented and is discussed in Chapter 5; however, the expense of educating high-level health care providers in Africa often prohibits expanding school enrollment. In Kenya, the cost of educating a single medical doctor from primary school to university is $65,997, and the cost of educating one nurse from primary school to college of health sciences is $43,180 (Kirigia et al., 2006). In addition to expense, a number of countries in Africa lack the indigenous capacity to produce enough physicians and must turn to medical training abroad for their students, who often opt not to return home to practice. This is especially true for the five Portuguese-speaking (Fronteira and Dussault, 2010; Villanueva, 2010) and war-torn countries in Africa (Crowe, 2005; Sillah, 2005). Those countries possessing the capacity to train may not have the absorptive capacity to expand their programs, which would require more teachers, more health facilities, and the ability to manage more programs.

Attempts are being made, however, to assist in improving and expanding medical education in Africa (NIH, 2010; SAMSS, 2010).

Training for HIV/AIDS Professional Support Staff

In addition to doctors and nurses, the HIV health workforce includes clinical officers, pharmacists, laboratory technicians, epidemiologists, phlebotomists, counselors, program managers, statisticians, data clerks, ancillary staff, and community health workers. The function of each category of health worker depends on the local model of care delivery and is influenced by tradition, legislation, and local regulations. Variation in health worker roles can be an obstacle to adapting generalized training tools and curricula to a specific setting (McCarthy et al., 2006).

Another category of health worker needed to respond to the HIV/AIDS epidemic in Africa consists of professional epidemiologists and other public health workers needed to manage and optimize health systems and the public's health. Unfortunately, there are critical gaps in advanced public health education in Africa (IJsselmuiden et al., 2007). On the continent as a whole, there are 29 countries without graduate public health training and 11 countries with only one such institution or program. Training is provided mainly by small units that lack the critical mass needed to expand the field of public health into the multisectoral effort it should be. The greatest shortages occur in lusophone and francophone Africa and in the one Spanish-speaking country (Equatorial Guinea). There are only 493 full-time faculty in public health for the entire continent (854 if part-time staff are counted as well). The overwhelming shortage of academic staff in public health in Africa is clear. While there is no clarity about an optimal number, fewer than 500 full-time academic staff distributed in small groups across Africa are unlikely to provide the public health leadership needed for nearly a billion people (IJsselmuiden et al., 2007).

Training for Less Specialized Workers

To respond to their human resource needs, African nations may be using or considering a health systems model that encourages the health workforce to share roles and responsibilities with other, less trained workers who can perform an aspect of HIV/AIDS care through task sharing (see Chapter 5). In May 2005, Family Health International's Zambia Prevention, Care and Treatment Partnership began training and placing community volunteers as lay counselors to complement the efforts of health workers in providing HIV counseling and help reduce their burden, using the national HIV counseling and testing curricula (Sanjana et al., 2009). This national training package includes a 2-week classroom component followed by a 4-week supervised practicum component. Utilizing a training system already in place in Africa could be a way of training less specialized workers in needed areas of HIV/AIDS prevention and treatment.

Technical and Vocational Education and Training (TVET)

Technical and vocational skills development has existed since the 1960s as a way of easing the problem of unemployment among primary school dropouts. In the last decade, such training has been gaining momentum in Africa, in large part as a result of evidence for its transformative role in East Asia and its continuing importance in Organisation for Economic Co-operation and Development countries (African Economic Outlook, 2010b). Students enrolled in formal TVET programs in Africa typically receive 3–6 years of training beyond primary school, depending on the country and the model. A recent survey conducted by the African Union on the state of TVET in 18 African countries suggests a number of priority areas for such training in Africa (African Union, 2007). The agricultural sector is of the highest priority, followed by public health and water resources, energy and environmental management, information and communication technologies, construction and maintenance, and good governance.

Although TVET could play a role in scaling up the supply of unskilled workers, enrollment in TVET programs in Africa remains marginal to poor. This low enrollment signals stagnation and overall inadequate public training capacity. Formal TVET is seriously underfunded, and obsolete equipment and weak managerial capacity affect the quality of programs. In addition, gender inequalities in TVET reflect the lower enrollment rates of women in secondary education generally (African Economic Outlook, 2010a).

The delivery of quality TVET depends in large part on the competence of teachers (African Union, 2007). Partnering with and learning from successful TVET programs in other African and non-African nations and utilizing twinning relationships as described in Chapter 5 could take advantage of a system already in place to develop the numbers and types of workers needed to respond to the challenges of scaling up HIV/AIDS services in Africa.

RECOMMENDATIONS

Recommendation 4-1: *Develop 10-year country roadmaps.* In parallel with the U.S. strategic planning called for in Recommendation 3-2, individual national HIV/AIDS coordinating bodies in Africa should develop, articulate, and update national 10-year roadmaps for combating HIV/AIDS. Each roadmap should take into account the implications of long-term projections of the national HIV/AIDS burden for institutions, communities, and resource requirements. As part of their roadmap, African governments should:

- invest sufficiently in HIV/AIDS prevention, following globally accepted best prevention practices;
- disclose national and subnational prevention outcomes and impacts and how they vary geographically and over time; and
- perform yearly evaluations to determine success as measured by change in HIV incidence data, as discussed in Recommendation 2-1.

Recommendation 4-2: *Develop and promote more efficient models of HIV/AIDS care and treatment.* African countries should invest in, evaluate, and apply more efficient models of HIV/AIDS care and treatment and promote those models through South–South learning exchanges.

Recommendation 4-3[2]: *Establish a governance contract.* African countries should establish a negotiated contract with U.S. agencies that includes programmatic targets and delineates each partner's responsibilities and expectations within a shared-responsibility approach. African governments should fully maintain the role and function of leadership and stewardship for policies and program implementation in their countries' health sector.

REFERENCES

Acemoglu, D., and S. Johnson. 2007. Disease and development: The effect of life expectancy on economic growth. *Journal of Political Economy* 115(6):925-983.

African Economic Outlook. 2010a. *Access to technical and vocational education in Africa.* http://www.africaneconomicoutlook.org/en/in-depth/developing-technical-and-vocational-skills-in-africa-2008/the-rationale-for-technical-and-vocational-skills-development/taking-stock-of-technical-and-vocational-skills-development/access-to-technical-and-vocational-education-in-africa/ (accessed October 29, 2010).

———. 2010b. *Brief history of the evolution of technical and vocational skills in national and international agendas.* http://www.africaneconomicoutlook.org/en/in-depth/developing-technical-and-vocational-skills-in-africa-2008/the-rationale-for-technical-and-vocational-skills-development/brief-history-of-the-evolution-of-technical-and-vocational-skills-in-national-and-international-agendas/ (accessed October 29, 2010).

African Union. 2007. Strategy to revitalize technical and vocational education and training (TVET) in Africa. Paper read at meeting of the Bureau of the Conference of Ministers of Education of the African Union (COMEDAF II+), Addis Ababa, Ethiopia.

Afrique Avenir. 2010. *World Bank donates mobile labs to Benin to fight HIV/AIDS.* http://www.afriqueavenir.org/en/2010/08/18/world-bank-donates-mobile-labs-to-benin-to-fight-hivaids/ (accessed August 26, 2010).

Ahmed, A. U., R. V. Hill, L. C. Smith, D. M. Wiesmann, T. Frankenberger, K. Gulati, W. Quabili, and Y. Yohannes. 2007. *The world's most deprived: Characteristics and causes of extreme poverty and hunger.* Washington, DC: International Food Policy Research Institute (IFPRI).

---

[2] See counterpart Recommendation 3-1 directed to the U.S. Office of the Global AIDS Coordinator.

Akwara, P. A., B. Noubary, P. Lim Ah Ken, K. Johnson, R. Yates, W. Winfrey, U. K. Chandan, D. Mulenga, J. Kolker, and C. Luo. 2010. Who is the vulnerable child? Using survey data to identify children at risk in the era of HIV and AIDS. *AIDS Care: Psychological and Socio-Medical Aspects of AIDS/HIV* 22(9):1066-1085.

Ansell, N., E. Robson, F. Hajdu, L. van Blerk, and L. Chipeta. 2009. The new variant famine hypothesis. *Progress in Development Studies* 9(3):187-207.

Arbache, J. S. 2009. Links between HIV/AIDS and development. In *The changing HIV/AIDS landscape: Selected papers for the World Bank's agenda for action in Africa, 2007-2011*, edited by E. L. Lule, R. M. Seifman, and A. C. David. Washington, DC: The World Bank. Pp. 63-79.

Arrehag, L., A. de Waal, and A. Whiteside. 2006. "New variant famine" revisited: Chronic vulnerability in rural Africa. *Humanitarian Exchange Magazine* 33:7-10.

Awases, M., A. Gbary, J. Nyoni, and R. Chatora. 2004. *Migration of health professionals in six countries: A synthesis report.* Geneva: WHO.

Ba, O., C. O'Regan, J. Nachega, C. Cooper, A. Anema, B. Rachlis, and E. J. Mills. 2008. HIV/AIDS in African militaries: An ecological analysis. *Medicine, Conflict, and Survival* 24(2):88-100.

Badri, M., D. Wilson, and R. Wood. 2002. Effect of highly active retroviral therapy on incidence of tuberculosis in South Africa: A cohort study. *The Lancet* 359:2059-2064.

Barks-Ruggles, E., T. Fantan, M. McPherson, and A. Whiteside. 2001. *Conference report: The economic impact of HIV/AIDS in southern Africa.* Washington, DC: The Brookings Institution.

Beard, J., F. Feeley, and S. Rosen. 2009. Economic and quality of life outcomes of antiretroviral therapy for HIV/AIDS in developing countries: A systematic literature review. *AIDS Care-Psychological and Socio-Medical Aspects of AIDS/HIV* 21(11):1343-1356.

Bedula, M., N. Ford, K. Hilderbrand, and H. Reuter. 2007. Implementing antiretroviral therapy in rural communities: The Lusikisiki model of decentralized HIV/AIDS care. *The Journal of Infectious Diseases* 196(Suppl. 3):S464-S468.

Bell, C., S. Devarajan, and H. Gersbach. 2004. Thinking about the long-run economic costs of AIDS. In *The macroeconomics of HIV/AIDS*, edited by M. Haacker. Washington, DC: The International Monetary Fund. Pp. 96-133.

Biesma, R. G., R. Brugha, A. Harmer, A. Walsh, N. Spicer, and G. Walt. 2009. The effects of global health initiatives on country health systems: A review of the evidence from HIV/AIDS control. *Health Policy and Planning* 24:239-252.

Bodibe, K. 2010. *South Africa: The link between mental health and HIV.* http://allafrica.com/stories/201009090505.html (accessed October 27, 2010).

Bodkin, C., H. Klopper, and G. Langley. 2006. A comparison of HIV positive and negative pregnant women at a public sector hospital in South Africa. *Journal of Clinical Nursing* 15(6):735-741.

Bolton-Moore, C., M. Mubiana-Mbewe, R. A. Cantrell, N. Chintu, E. M. Stringer, B. H. Chi, M. Sinkala, C. Kankasa, C. M. Wilson, C. M. Wilfert, A. Mwango, J. Levy, E. J. Abrams, M. Bulterys, and J. S. A. Stringer. 2007. Clinical outcomes and CD4 cell response in children receiving antiretroviral therapy at primary health care facilities in Zambia. *Journal of the American Medical Association* 298(16):1888-1899.

Booysen, F. 2004a. Income and poverty dynamics in HIV/AIDS-affected households in the free state province of South Africa. *South African Journal of Economics* 72:522-545.

———. 2004b. Social grants as safety net for HIV/AIDS-affected households in South Africa. *SAHARA J: Journal of Social Aspects of HIV/AIDS Research Alliance/SAHARA/Human Sciences Research Council* 1(1):45-56.

Boulle, A., and N. Ford. 2007. Scaling up antiretroviral therapy in developing countries: What are the benefits and challenges? *Sexually Transmitted Infections* 83:503-505.

Candiani, T. M., P. Jorge, C. A. Araújo Cardoso, M. Carneiro, and E. A. Goulart. 2007. Impact of highly active antiretroviral therapy (HAART) on the incidence of opportunistic infections, hospitalizations and mortality among children and adolescents living with HIV/AIDS in Belo Horizonte, Minas Gerais State, Brazil. *Cadernos de saúde pública/Ministério da Saúde, Fundação Oswaldo Cruz, Escola Nacional de Saúde Pública* 23(Suppl. 3):S414-S423.

Cates, W. J., and A. R. Hinman. 1992. AIDS and absolutism—The demand for perfection in prevention. *The New England Journal of Medicine* 327(7):492-494.

Chirambo, K. 2009. The impact of HIV/AIDS on the electoral process in Namibia, Malawi, Senegal, South Africa, Tanzania and Zambia. In *Governance of HIV/AIDS: Making participation and accountability count*, edited by S. Harman and F. Lisk. London: Routledge. Pp. 11-34.

Cohen, M., and C. Gay. 2010. Treatment to prevent transmission of HIV-1. *Clinical Infectious Diseases* 50(Suppl. 3):S85-S95.

Commission on HIV/AIDS and Governance in Africa. 2008. *Securing our future: Report of the Commission on HIV/AIDS and Governance in Africa.* http://www.uneca.org/CHGA/Report/CHGAReport.pdf (accessed October 29, 2010).

Coovadia, H., and R. Bland. 2008. From Alma-Ata to Agincourt: Primary health care in AIDS. *The Lancet* 372:866-868.

Creese, A., K. Floyd, A. Alban, and L. Guinness. 2002. Cost-effectiveness of HIV/AIDS interventions in Africa: A systematic review of the evidence. *The Lancet* 359(9318):1635-1642.

Crowe, S. 2005. Angola: After 30 years of civil war, school reconstruction helps build a bright future. *UNICEF-Newsline*, July 28, 2005.

Crush, J., B. Frayne, and M. Grant. 2006. *Linking migration, HIV/AIDS and urban food security in southern and eastern Africa.* http://programs.ifpri.org/renewal/pdf/UrbanRural.pdf (accessed November 1, 2010).

Csáky, C. 2009. *Keeping children out of harmful institutions: Why we should be investing in family-based care.* London: Save the Children.

de-Graft Aikins, A., N. Unwin, C. Agyemang, P. Allotey, C. Campbell, and D. Arhinful. 2010. Tackling Africa's chronic disease burden: From the local to the global. *Globalization and Health* 6(1):5.

De Maeseneer, J., C. van Weel, D. Egilman, K. Mfenyana, A. Kaufman, N. Sewankambo, and M. Flinkenflögel. 2008. Funding for primary health care in developing countries: Money from disease specific projects could be used to strengthen primary care. *British Medical Journal* 336:518-519.

de Waal, A. 2003. How will HIV/AIDS transform African governance? *African Affairs* 102:1-23.

———. 2007. The politics of a health crisis: Why AIDS is not threatening African governance. *Harvard International Review* 20-24.

———. 2010. Reframing governance, security and conflict in the light of HIV/AIDS: A synthesis of findings from AIDS, security and conflict initiative. *Social Science and Medicine* 70:114-120.

de Waal, A., and A. Whiteside. 2003. New variant famine: AIDS and food crisis in southern Africa. *The Lancet* 362(9391):1234-1237.

Desmond, C., and J. Gow. 2001. *The cost-effectiveness of six models of care for orphan and vulnerable children in South Africa.* Durban University of Natal-Health Economics and HIV/AIDS Research Division.

Dionne, K. Y., P. Gerland, and S. Watkins. 2008. AIDS exceptionalism: The view from below. In *Malawi longitudinal study of families and health, wave 5.* Philadelphia: University of Pennsylvania.

Drimie, S., and M. Casale. 2009. Multiple stressors in southern Africa: The link between HIV/AIDS, food security, poverty and children's vulnerability now and in the future. *AIDS Care* 21(Suppl. 1):S28-S33.

Duber, H., T. J. Coates, G. Szekeres, A. H. Kaji, and R. J. Lewis. 2010. Is there an association between PEPFAR funding and improvement in national health indicators in Africa? A retrospective study. *Journal of the International AIDS Society* 13:21.

Eboko, F. 2005. *Patterns of mobilization: Political culture in the fight against AIDS.* Edited by A. S. Patterson. Hants, England: Ashgate. Pp. 37-58.

Embrey, M., D. Hoos, and J. Quick. 2009. How AIDS funding strengthens health systems: Progress in pharmaceutical management. *Journal of Acquired Immune Deficiency Syndromes* 52(Suppl. 1):S34-S37.

Feeley, F. G. III, S. Rosen, and P. J. Connelly. 2009. The private sector and HIV/AIDS in Africa: Recent developments and implications for policy. In *The changing HIV/AIDS landscape: Selected papers for the World Bank's agenda for action in Africa, 2007-2011*, edited by E. L. Lule, R. M. Seifman, and A. C. David. Washington, DC: The World Bank. Pp. 267-293.

Ford, N., E. Mills, and A. Calmy. 2009. Rationing antiretroviral therapy in Africa—Treating too few, too late. *The New England Journal of Medicine* 360(18):1808-1810.

Forster, M., C. Bailey, M. W. Brinkhof, C. Graber, A. Boulle, M. Spohr, E. Balestre, M. May, O. Keiser, A. Jahn, and M. Egger. 2008. Electronic medical record systems, data quality and loss to follow-up: Survey of antiretroviral therapy programmes in resource-limited settings. *Bulletin of the World Health Organization* 86(12):939-947.

Frayne, B. 2006. HIV/AIDS and rural food security in Africa: Discussion. *Review of Agricultural Economics* 25(3):458-460.

Freedman, L. P. 2005. Achieving the MDGs: Health systems as core social institutions. *Development* 48(1):19.

Freeman, M., N. Nkomo, Z. Kafaar, and K. Kelly. 2007. Factors associated with prevalence of mental disorder in people living with HIV/AIDS in South Africa. *AIDS Care: Psychological and Socio-medical Aspects of AIDS/HIV* 19(10):1201-1209.

Fronteira, I., and G. Dussault. 2010. Human resources in the health sector of Portuguese-speaking African countries: Identical problems, cross-sectional solutions? *Electronic Journal of Communication, Information & Innovation in Health (RECIIS)* 4(1):71-78.

Gebo, K., J. Fleishman, and R. Moore. 2005. Hospitalizations for metabolic conditions, opportunistic infections, and injection drug use among HIV patients: Trends between 1996 and 2000 in 12 states. *Journal of Acquired Immune Deficiency Syndromes* 40(5):609-616.

Gill, T. B. 2010. Modeling the impact of HIV/AIDS upon food security of diverse rural households in western Kenya. *Agricultural Systems* 103(5):265-281.

Gimbel-Sherr, S. O., M. A. Micek, K. H. Gimbel-Sherr, T. Koepsell, J. P. Hughes, K. K. Thomas, J. Pfeiffer, and S. S. Gloyd. 2007. Using nurses to identify HAART eligible patients in the Republic of Mozambique: Results of a time series analysis. *Human Resources for Health* 5(7):1-9.

Greener, R. 2004. The impact of HIV/AIDS on poverty and inequality. In *The macroeconomics of HIV/AIDS*, edited by M. Haacker. Washington, DC: The International Monetary Fund. Pp. 167-181.

Haacker, M. 2006. Fiscal and macroeconomic aspects of the HIV pandemic. In *The HIV pandemic—Local and global implications*, edited by E. Beck. New York: Oxford University Press.

———. 2009. Impact of and response to HIV/AIDS: Public policy challenges. In *The changing HIV/AIDS landscape: Selected papers for the World Bank's agenda for action in Africa, 2007-2011*, edited by E. L. Lule, R. M. Seifman, and A. C. David. Washington, DC: The World Bank. Pp. 197-225.

Habyarimana, J., B. Mbakile, and C. Pop-Eleches. 2010. The impact of HIV/AIDS and ARV treatment on worker absenteeism: Implications for African firms. *Journal of Human Resources* 45(4):809-839.

Hagopian, A., M. Thompson, M. Fordyce, K. Johnson, and L. G. Hart. 2004. The migration of physicians from sub-Saharan Africa to the United States of America: Measures of the African brain drain. *Human Resources for Health* 2(1):17.

Harling, G., C. Orrell, and R. Wood. 2007. Healthcare utilization of patients accessing an African national treatment program. *BMC Health Services Research* 7.

Harman, S. 2009. The causes, contours and consequences of the multisectoral response to HIV/AIDS. In *Governance of HIV/AIDS: Making participation and accountability count*, edited by S. Harman and F. Lisk. London: Routledge. Pp. 163-179.

Harman, S., and F. Lisk, eds. 2009. *Governance of the HIV/AIDS response: Making participation and accountability count*. London: Routledge.

WHO, UNAIDS, and UNICEF. 2009. *Towards universal access: Scaling up priority HIV/AIDS interventions in the health sector: Progress report 2009.* Geneva: WHO.

———. 2010. *Towards universal access: Scaling up priority HIV/AIDS interventions in the health sector: Progress report 2010.* Geneva: WHO.

Wilson, D., and S. Challa. 2009. HIV epidemiology: Recent trends and lessons. In *The changing HIV/AIDS landscape: Selected papers for the World Bank's agenda for action in Africa, 2007-2011*, edited by E. L. Lule, R. M. Seifman, and A. C. David. Washington, DC: The World Bank. Pp. 7-28.

Wong, M. H., K. Robertson, N. Nakasujja, R. Skolasky, S. Musisi, E. Katabira, J. C. McArthur, A. Ronald, and N. Sacktor. 2007. Frequency of and risk factors for HIV dementia in an HIV clinic in sub-Saharan Africa. *Neurology* 68(5):350-355.

World Bank and International Monetary Fund. 2008. *Global monitoring report. MDGs and the environment: Agenda for inclusive and sustainable development.* Washington, DC: World Bank.

World Bank and USAID. 2010 (unpublished). *Test and treat: Can we treat our way out of the HIV epidemic.* Washington, DC: World Bank and USAID.

Young, C. 1994. *The African colonial state in comparative perspective.* New Haven, CT: Yale University Press.

Yu, D., Y. Souteyrand, M. Banda, J. Kaufman, and J. Perriens. 2008. Investment in HIV/AIDS programs: Does it help strengthen health systems in developing countries? *Globalization and Health* 4(1):8.

5

Strategies to Build Capacity for Prevention, Treatment, and Care of HIV/AIDS in Africa

Key Findings

- Given increasing numbers of patients, shortages of trained medical personnel, and financial constraints, there is a need to provide treatment and services for HIV/AIDS more efficiently.
- Governments and nongovernmental organizations in Africa can build additional capacity for prevention, treatment, and care of HIV/AIDS by making the most of existing capacities. They can accomplish this by employing appropriate staffing models to optimize impact and utilizing the capacity of local institutions.
- The United States and other donor countries can play a role in building institutional and human resource capacity to prepare for the long-term burden of HIV/AIDS in Africa by supporting partnerships at all levels, as well as other capacity-building programs.

This chapter describes a variety of strategies to build capacity[1] for prevention, treatment, and care of HIV/AIDS in Africa. Strategies for African governments and institutions as well as the United States (and other donor nations) are explored. First, however, the chapter provides a context for these strategies by briefly reviewing the present state of human resources for health care in Africa.

---

[1] The term *capacity building* is used to describe an initiative in which an organization engages in enhancing a partner's human, scientific, technological, organizational, institutional, and/or resource capabilities (UNCED, 1992).

PRESENT STATE OF HUMAN RESOURCES
FOR HEALTH CARE IN AFRICA

As discussed in Chapter 1, current resource constraints in donor nations and the growing HIV-related needs and demand for treatment in Africa are at odds. Lacking well-functioning health systems,[2] African nations are ill prepared to confront the looming HIV/AIDS burden of 2020 to 2025. Accordingly, the international community must focus on enabling them to muster the necessary internal resources. A major requirement to this end is to strengthen health care systems, in particular by building institutional and human resource capacity.

The Health Workforce Crisis

Health workforces play a crucial role in achieving the United Nations' Millennium Development Goals (MDGs). For example, the supply of health workers impacts the health of women and children. Yet only 5 of 49 low-income countries have the minimum 23 doctors per 10,000 inhabitants, recommended by the World Health Organization (WHO) (WHO, 2010a). Three major forces challenge the health workforce in Africa. First is the devastation of HIV/AIDS, increasing workloads, exposing workers to infection, and trying their morale. Second is accelerating labor migration, causing losses of nurses and doctors from countries that can least afford the "brain drain." Third is the legacy of chronic underinvestment in human resources; frozen recruitment and salaries; and restricted public budgets, depleting work environments of basic supplies, drugs, and facilities (JLI, 2004). Continued underinvestment in the health care workforce is detrimental to staff morale and the ethos of care.

In addition to health workers being compensated insufficiently and asked to work under harsh conditions with few supplies and little support, an extreme imbalance exists in the distribution of credentialed health professionals among regions and countries (and by geographic location within the same country). The problem of insufficient human resources for health care is particularly acute in Africa, which bears 25 percent of the world's burden of disease but is home to only 1.3 percent of the world's health workforce (Commission for Africa, 2005; High-Level Forum on the Health MDGs, 2004). Currently, an estimated 750,000 health workers serve the 682 million people of sub-Saharan Africa, representing an extremely low health care provider-to-population ratio; by comparison, the ratio is 10 to 15 times higher in Organisation for Economic Co-operation and Development (OECD) countries (see Figure 5-1) (High-Level Forum on the Health MDGs, 2004).

---

[2] As defined by WHO, a functioning health system should include access to adequate financing; essential medical products, vaccines, and technologies; a well-performing health workforce; reliable and timely health information; and strategic policy frameworks to provide effective analysis, oversight, and governance (WHO, 2007a).

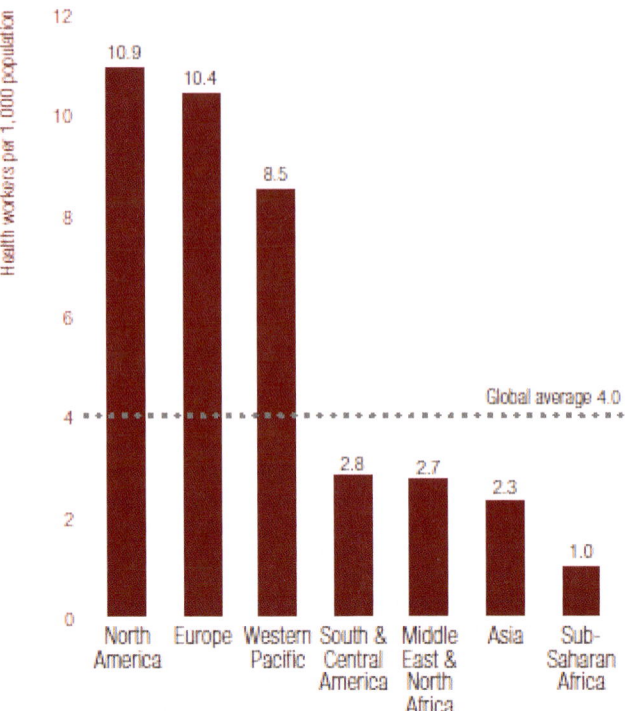

FIGURE 5-1 Health worker density by region.
SOURCE: JLI, 2004, compiled from WHO, 2004.

Any efforts to stabilize and improve health in the region must address this shortage of human resources for health care. Health care services cannot be delivered in the absence of a viable workforce. Any sustainable solution to Africa's health problems will require a stable cadre of medical officers, nurses, clinical officers,[3] dentists, and allied health workers—not only as clinicians, but also as teachers, managers, and leaders. A 2005 analysis of the human resource requirements of the U.S. President's Emergency Plan for AIDS Relief (PEPFAR) found that providing even 90 minutes of physician time per year to each of the 2 million patients on antiretroviral therapy (ART) would require about 20 percent or more of the existing physician workforce in 5 of the 14 PEPFAR countries (Ethiopia, Mozambique, Rwanda, Tanzania, and Zambia). The severity of the

---

[3] In Africa, medical officers are the equivalent of a physician and have graduated from medical school. Clinical officers have 3-4 years of post–high school education and are able to perform their duties with a fair amount of independence.

human resource shortage was found to vary widely; some countries are much better positioned for a rapid scale-up of services than others (IOM, 2005c). The training of the necessary cadre of health workers, prepared and supported to confront their countries' health issues, is a key challenge that all African nations must face (SAMSS, 2010).

The Lack of Education and Training

Educational systems of developing countries are a major impediment to the ongoing production and retention of health workers. Europe produces 173,800 physicians a year and Africa only 5,100 (see Figure 5-2) (Chen et al., 2004; JLI, 2004). One physician is produced for every 5,000 people in Central and Eastern

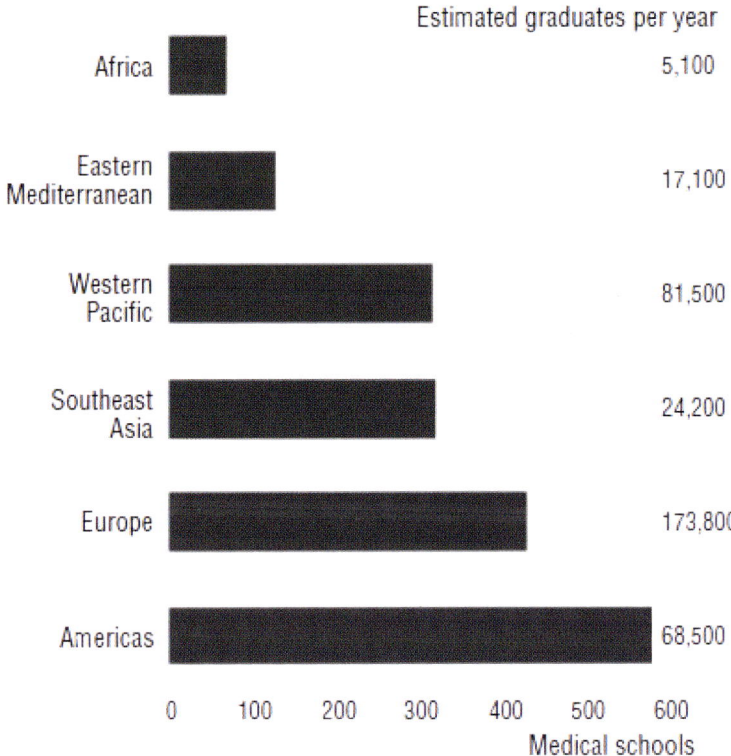

FIGURE 5-2 Regional disparities in numbers of medical schools and graduates.
NOTE: "Region" refers to World Health Organization (WHO) regions.
SOURCE: Eckhert, 2002; JLI, 2004.

Europe and the Baltic States, compared with one for every 115,000 people in Africa (IOM, 2005a). Similarly, the output of nurses in Africa lags far behind that in economically developed countries of the world. In 2005, for example, Cape Verde had only 100 nursing school graduates and Mozambique just 128, while in 2006, Guinea Bissau had only 62 (WHO, 2010b). The United States has one nurse for every 125 people, while Uganda has one nurse for every 5,000 people. And in all of Rwanda, there are only 11 pharmacists (IOM, 2005a).

Universities in low-income countries often face a number of challenges in meeting the need to educate and train the health workforce, including a lack of funds, weak infrastructure, outdated or misaligned training programs, overcrowded classrooms, and overburdened and underpaid staff (Dovlo, 2003; Tettey, 2006). For students in training, the shortage of teachers translates into little mentorship or academic support. Health program graduates are often ill equipped to perform the critical tasks for which they are needed and are unprepared to deal with the challenges of working in underresourced hospitals and clinics (IOM, 2009; Taché et al., 2008; WHO, 2006). The overall lack of opportunity and career advancement results in low morale, providing little incentive to work in academia or the public sector, or even to remain in the country (IOM, 2009).

STRATEGIES TO BUILD CAPACITY FOR PREVENTION, TREATMENT, AND CARE OF HIV/AIDS IN AFRICA

Governments and nongovernmental organizations in the United States and other donor countries and within Africa can help build capacity for prevention, treatment, and care of HIV/AIDS in Africa. This section details the gaps to be filled by partnering and the structures, systems, and professions necessary to implement partnerships and other capacity-building strategies, and describes promising strategies that can be implemented now by African nations and the United States to prepare for the long-term burden of HIV/AIDS in Africa.

Gaps to Be Filled by Partnering

Projects made possible through partnerships, including "twinning,"[4] can fill a variety of gaps in current HIV/AIDS prevention, treatment, and care programs. With respect to teaching, for example, partnerships increase access to faculty experts currently in short supply in Africa. Partnerships can also:

---

[4] The Interagency Coalition on AIDS and Development defines twinning as a collaboration between two or more organizations that must be formal—including an agreement or contract—and substantive—meaning the interaction spans a period of time beyond a one-time knowledge- or service-seeking interaction (ICAD, 2002; Vian et al., 2007). In the context of this study, twinning is defined as a bilateral, mutually beneficial capacity-building partnership formed to mitigate the effects of HIV/AIDS in Africa.

- facilitate the introduction of new, cutting-edge technologies for laboratories, informatics, logistics, communications, and teaching through training by partners more familiar with these innovations;
- provide a consultation network offering access to high-level technical consultants for patient care in such areas as clinical care, pathology, radiography, and public health;
- facilitate access to relatively rare clinical services, such as reference laboratory support for anatomic or clinical pathology (e.g., pathologic diagnosis of complications of HIV/AIDS);
- enable electronic sharing of curricula and library resources;
- provide access to professional development to improve the teaching ability of faculty;
- assist in developing grant management capacities to enable African institutions to obtain support for operations research and evaluation;
- provide training in operations research; and
- provide resources to strengthen the entire health system, not just clinical services.

Structures, Systems, and Professions Necessary to Implement Partnerships and Other Capacity-Building Strategies

The objectives of HIV/AIDS partnerships depend on both the needs and interests of the host country and the resources available to the partner organizations. Careful consideration of the partners' basic capacity is essential for sustainable and mutually beneficial partnerships. Each organization involved must have at least the minimum institutional capacity (including staff, capital, infrastructure, and funding) necessary to support the scope of the planned partnership (ICAD, 1999). If staffing is already stretched thin at one or both of the organizations prior to partnering, the endeavor should be reconsidered. Table 5-1 lists the common types of partnerships for capacity building.

Additionally, it is crucially important for the partners to engage within not only the cultural and contextual reality but also the governmental and national planning framework of the host country, as well as to coordinate with other organizations on the ground. Successful capacity building supports national health plans and health system development and is fundamentally based in and guided and led by host country partners—particularly since government capacity is itself crucial to the future course of the African HIV/AIDS epidemic.

Promising Strategies for Highly Affected Nations in Africa: Making the Most of Existing Capacities

Governments and nongovernmental organizations within Africa can build additional capacity for prevention, treatment, and care of HIV/AIDS by making

TABLE 5-1 The Partnership Continuum

Type of Partnership	Description
Short-term consultation/technical assistance	A partnership involving the transfer of knowledge or skills from an organization in a developed, donor country to individual employees working for a partner organization in a developing country (Jensen et al., 2007). This transfer of knowledge and skills is accomplished through the provision of physical infrastructure (buildings, vehicles, and equipment), formal education and consultation, and training of staff at large (Jones and Blunt, 1999).
Individual to individual	A partnership involving training, coaching, and mentoring from an experienced individual to a less experienced individual through on-site shadowing, site visits, or telephone/Internet consultation (McCarthy et al., 2006).
Institution to institution • Universities • Health care institutions • National academies • Public health institutes • Regional/compact bodies • Professional organizations • Civil society and nongovernmental organizations • Faith-based organizations	A long-term collaboration between two organizations. Institutional partnerships are the basis for familiar, long-term relationships in which the partners share values and experiences (Dada et al., 2009).
Government to government	A partnering of national governments or subsets and agencies thereof, such as ministries of health, for the purpose of leadership strengthening and information sharing. These partnerships encourage effective "discharge [of the host country's] responsibilities for stewardship and governance of country-level health systems" (Omaswa and Ivey Boufford, 2010) (Foreword).

the most of existing capacities. This section highlights promising strategies that can be used to this end. These strategies fall into two broad categories: employing appropriate staffing models to optimize impact and utilizing the capacity of local institutions.

Appropriate Staffing Models to Optimize Impact

In many settings, HIV/AIDS prevention, treatment, and care are provided through complex, overburdened delivery systems that require specialist physicians. Yet many in need of these services live in rural settings, far from specialized care. To illustrate the point, Figure 5-3 shows that 67 percent of the cost of treatment is not for medication, but for the systems used to deliver it to patients and maintain them on it (UNAIDS, 2010a,b). Given increasing numbers of patients, shortages of trained medical personnel, and financial constraints, there is a need to provide services for HIV/AIDS more efficiently (UNAIDS, 2010b). The committee identified a number of strategies that could be implemented to achieve this goal: use of management and support staff, task sharing, harnessing of the informal health sector, use of modern information technology, analytic planning for the health workforce, and investment in women as health workers.

Management and support staff The 2008 Kampala Declaration and Agenda for Global Action recommended that "governments, civil society, [the] private sector, and professional organizations [work together] to strengthen leadership and management capacity at all levels" (WHO, 2008a). In addition to health care professionals, scale-up of HIV/AIDS prevention, treatment, and care programs must rely heavily on personnel from outside the clinical health sector who can

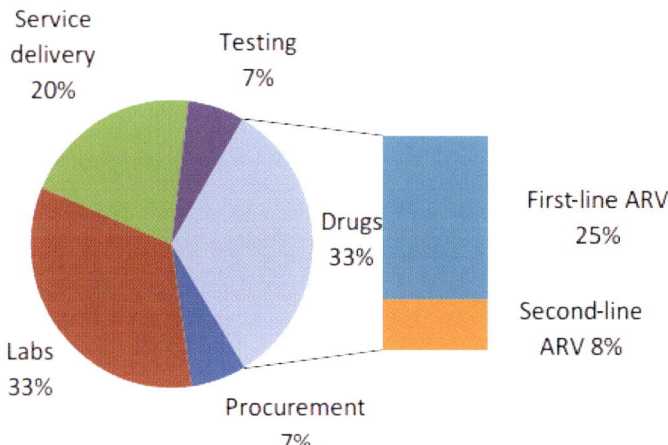

FIGURE 5-3 Breakdown of HIV/AIDS treatment costs in low- and middle-income countries.
NOTE: ARV = antiretroviral drug.
SOURCE: UNAIDS, 2010a.

TABLE 5-2 Imbalance in Health Worker Ratios

WHO Region	Percentage of Total Health Workforce		
	Health Service Provider	Health Management and Support	Ratio
Africa	83	17	4.9:1
Eastern Mediterranean	75	25	3.0:1
South East Asia	67	33	2.0:1
Western Pacific	78	23	3.4:1
Europe	69	31	2.7:1
Americas	57	43	1.3:1
The World	67	33	2.0:1

SOURCE: Dare, 2010. Adapted from WHO, 2006.

free up time for health care providers to perform clinical work. For example, laboratory technicians can play an essential role in the administration and monitoring of ART. Other types of personnel with needed competencies include, for example, nutritionists; counselors; behavioral specialists; management personnel; information technologists; procurement and distribution professionals; drug regulatory professionals; data analysts; and experts in monitoring, evaluation, and operations research.

Furthermore, it is important that management and support functions be performed by personnel with expertise in those roles and not by clinical service providers, whose time is much better spent attending to medical matters. Yet as Table 5-2 shows, there is a global imbalance in health worker ratios. In the Americas, the ratio of clinical service providers to management and support staff is almost 1:1; in Africa, that ratio is almost 5:1 (Dare, 2010; WHO, 2006). A considerable increase in clinical care could be delivered without adding more clinicians if the management and support capacity of others in HIV/AIDS prevention, treatment, and care were increased.

Task sharing Sharing of roles and responsibilities is not a new concept in the provision of health care; realignment of roles and responsibilities has been a long-standing response to changing health care needs, particularly in emergency situations or underserved areas.[5] As a result of the HIV/AIDS crisis, the concept has reemerged with increased urgency. One term used to describe shared or realigned responsibilities is "task shifting." WHO defines task shifting as

---

[5] In fact, what is sometimes understood as realignment of roles is actually formal recognition of the contributions of health workers that have previously been "invisible." For example, midwives were important providers of obstetrical services even before physician involvement in obstetrical care, but may now be seen as having "inherited" this responsibility from physicians as their roles have become more prominent.

the process whereby specific tasks are transferred, when appropriate, to health workers with less training and fewer qualifications (WHO, 2008c). Although this term does not adequately encompass the concepts of realignment and recognition of appropriate responsibility, it does capture a narrower and sometimes temporary arrangement to meet emergency needs. The underlying assumption is that shifting specific tasks enables more efficient use of existing human resources and eases bottlenecks in service delivery. When additional human resources are needed, task shifting may also involve the delegation of some clearly delineated tasks to newly created cadres of health workers who receive specific competency-based training (WHO, 2008c).

The delegation of the health care responsibilities of nurses, physicians, clinical officers, dentists, and other health professionals to others, including community health workers, has been effective in addressing the severe human resource shortages in many African countries (Buchan and Poz, 2003; Glenngård and Anell, 2003; Morris et al., 2009). Because these responsibilities require not only skills but also relevant knowledge, this delegation goes beyond the mere performance of specific tasks. The committee has therefore elected to use the term "task sharing" rather than "task shifting" in this report. Task sharing that is needs-based, is not hierarchical or territorial, and allows roles to expand or contract according to need is the most appropriate approach to health care delivery in low-resource environments.

Health workers who are normally viewed as auxiliary are increasingly becoming the main providers of health services in many countries. In Africa, for example, nurse aids, medical assistants, and clinical officers are performing essential medical tasks, especially in rural areas. A good example is Malawi, where clinical officers are a major resource, performing surgical procedures and administering anesthesia, as well as providing medical care (Hongoro and McPake, 2004).

Another example is South Africa, where the unprecedented challenges of people requiring care and treatment for HIV/AIDS are forcing a rethinking and reorganization of health resources and health systems and a reappraisal of the role of nurses in care for complex and chronic illnesses. South Africa's health system has historically been nurse driven, and nurses outnumber physicians five to one. Yet while the majority of the population receives formal health care from nurses rather than doctors, it is clear that nurses have been insufficiently empowered, resourced, and compensated to carry out their key roles effectively (Dohrn et al., 2009). Developing HIV/AIDS expertise among nurses has become a national priority, as is illustrated in South Africa's National HIV/AIDS Strategic Plan (South African Department of Health, 2006). Accordingly, the South African Department of Health initiated new certificate courses in prevention of mother-to-child transmission (PMTCT) and ART for nurses in 2002 (Dohrn et al., 2009). The new "PMTCT nurses" and "ART nurses" are the unofficial gatekeepers of HIV/AIDS knowledge and skills at the primary health care level.

They direct HIV testing and counseling services, prepare patients for ART initiation, diagnose and manage side effects and opportunistic infections, partner with midwives to provide PMTCT services during the perinatal period, and provide early infant diagnostic services. They are trained to refer patients ready for ART initiation and those with advanced illness and complications (Dohrn et al., 2009; Morris et al., 2009).

A recent randomized controlled trial in South Africa compared nurse and physician management of HIV-infected patients receiving ART at two South African primary care clinics and found that primary health nurses were noninferior to doctors in monitoring of first-line ART (Sanne et al., 2010). The inclusion of PMTCT and ART initiation programs in health service basic training programs within African institutions of higher education (rather than during in-service training) could alleviate much of the need for posteducation in-service training and prepare graduates who can enter the workforce capable of initiating and managing ART and related complications.

The expansion of the numbers and roles of auxiliaries whose qualifications are not internationally recognized appears to be a quiet success story, providing large numbers of health workers who keep the system running in a number of countries (Hongoro and McPake, 2004). These alternatives are worth investigating given that there is a long lead time to increase the health care workforce. Depending on the type of degree and the specific country, the amount of training required can vary. For example, in South Africa it takes 4 years to train nursing or midwife students, 2 years to train pupil nurses, and 1 year to train pupil nursing auxiliaries (South African Nursing Council, 2010). By contrast, in Mozambique basic nurses are educated to grade 10 and have an additional 18 months of training; medium nurses are also educated to grade 10, but receive an additional two and a half years of training thereafter; and superior nurses are educated through grade 12 and must graduate from a 4-year university with a baccalaureate degree (August-Brady, 2010). As with nurses, the amount of training required for physicians varies by country. In Mozambique it takes a medical student 7 years to attain a medical degree (Ferrinho et al., 2010). In South Africa, medical school courses last 5 years (University of KwaZulu-Natal, 2010), followed by 2 years of internship and 1 year of community service, for a total requirement of 8 years to become a practicing physician.

Task sharing may not be readily accepted by various professions. Physicians and pharmacists have objected to the delegation of their tasks to those whom they perceive as professionals with less specialized training, while nurses have resisted taking on physicians' roles without commensurate salary increases. Policies to enable task sharing, such as remuneration packages and clear job descriptions and strategic plans delineating professional boundaries and responsibilities, need to be established (Zachariah et al., 2009). The pivotal issue for the sustainability of task sharing will be how governments and international and bilateral organizations help prepare health systems to implement the practice, develop adequate understanding of existing capacity, and make full use of existing roles and personnel. African government regulations supportive of task sharing would help optimize the impact of heath care workers in low-resource contexts. National governments also must garner the support of the various stakeholders who affect and are affected by the reconfiguration of tasks (such as professional bodies and associations; trade unions; ministries of health, education, finance, and public service; nongovernmental and community organizations; and local health structures). Otherwise, task sharing will exist on the political and organizational periphery of the formal health system; be exposed to shifts in policy and funding; and become fragile and unsustainable, further depleting a demoralized health system.

Harnessing of the informal health sector Home-based care of patients is becoming increasingly important in many societies, particularly where health facilities are overwhelmed by HIV/AIDS, and patients are returned to their homes to be cared for or await death (Omaswa, 2006). The care provided in the home by unpaid and untrained family members and friends and neighbors of those living with HIV/AIDS is not linked with any formal care or support services.[6] Up to 90 percent of care for the ill is provided by this unlinked system of home care (Ogden et al., 2004; Uys, 2003). This care is provided primarily by women and is largely overlooked in both governmental and nongovernmental efforts to mitigate the impact of the epidemic (Ogden et al., 2004).

In a number of African countries with high HIV/AIDS prevalence, overburdened health systems, and a lack of resources (including hospital beds and health workers), the option of treating HIV/AIDS patients at home can be attractive to governments (Avert, 2010). One South African hospital reported that patients' average stay decreased from 14 days to 3.5 days when they were referred to a home-based care organization (Fox et al., 2002). Home-based community care allows clinics and hospitals to minimize patient admissions; lowers the costs of health services and hospitalizations; and alleviates the pressures on clinic and hospital staff, enabling them to serve other clients (Ogden et al., 2004).

In addition to unlinked home-based care, a significant proportion of health care is provided in commercial settings such as markets, shops, and elsewhere in many African communities. Vendors are regularly called upon to advise purchasers on the effects of the health products they sell and how the products should be used. In many cases, these merchants and shopkeepers interview buyers, take medical histories, and proceed to diagnose and prescribe. Where formal health care facilities are not easily accessed, this group of informal health workers is the first and most important point of call for people in search of health services (Omaswa, 2006).

It is estimated that some 70 percent of Africans access traditional healers

---

[6] In comparison, "linked" home-based care refers to care (clinical and nonclinical) that is provided by lay, volunteer, or professional providers who are linked to formal programs (Ogden et al., 2004).

(Mills et al., 2006). In rural South Africa, over 60 percent of the population seeks health advice and treatment from traditional healers before visiting a physician (AMREF, 2010). Thus, the strategy of partnering with traditional healers and bringing them into the formal health system should be considered. Indeed, rather than ostracizing traditional healers, WHO has advocated for their inclusion in national HIV/AIDS programs since the early 1990s; in 1994, WHO suggested upgrading traditional healers' skills rather than training a new cadre of health workers (UNAIDS, 2000). In the future, it may be important to provide forums where biomedical practitioners and traditional healers can share experiences and be trained together so they can become sources of mutual referral.

Informal health workers are found in every health system, and the impact of their role increases as the strength of the formal sector weakens. Unlinked health care providers—such as those providing home-based care, informal drug vendors, and traditional healers—play important roles in some communities and deserve to be acknowledged, encouraged, and supported (Omaswa, 2006).

Use of modern information technology Recent advances have resulted in a dramatic increase in the use of information and communication technology (ICT) applications in health care, collectively known as "e-Health" (WHO, 2010c). e-Health applications, including teleconsultations, telereferrals, forward-storage concepts (e.g., teleradiology and teleprescriptions), and electronic patient records, can directly support training of community health workers, prevention, patient diagnosis, and patient management and care (WHO, 2007b).

Cellular and smart phones, for example, can be used to increase the efficiency of overburdened health workers, extending their reach by overcoming barriers of distance and time. Box 5-1 provides examples of how smart phone technology is being used to improve case management and drug tracking. Modern ICT can also facilitate distance learning. Web-based or electronic applications can deliver training to health workers on an asynchronous (i.e., not in real time) and independent basis. Such distance learning models offer cost savings because they do not require dedicated lecturers or administrators, nor do they incur travel or lodging expenses or require trainees to spend time away from their jobs (Accordia Global Health Foundation, 2010). In addition to these technologies, clinical teaching labs with simulation mannequins for self-teaching of clinical skills, as well as computerized scenarios and self-teaching guides, could be considered for training the African health care workforce.

Analytic planning for the health workforce The 2008 Kampala Declaration and Agenda for Global Action called for governments to "determine the appropriate health workforce skill mix" and "create health workforce information systems, to improve research and to develop capacity for data management in order to institutionalize evidence-based decision-making and enhance shared learning" (WHO, 2008a, pp. 10–11). Similarly, the 2010 World Health Assembly encour-

---

BOX 5-1
Smart Phones for Health Worker Efficiency:
eMOCHA and SmartTrack

eMOCHA is a free open-source application developed by the Johns Hopkins Center for Clinical Global Health Education. It is designed to assist health programs in developing countries in improving provider communication, education, and patient care by coordinating wireless devices with local server-based clinical training and patient care support services (eMOCHA, 2010). eMOCHA combines the power of wireless mobile collection of patient data and the capacity of the new Android-supported devices to display high-quality interactive touch screen forms, as well as video and audio files, with the power of server-based applications. These capabilities make it possible to analyze and map large amounts of data from the community and to create new training content in a variety of formats (eMOCHA, 2010).

SmartTrack is another example of how cellular phones can assist with the management of HIV/AIDS programs. SmartTrack is a telehealth project aimed at addressing the problem of theft and counterfeiting of HIV/AIDS medications. The goal is to create a highly reliable, secure, and ultra-low-cost cell phone–based distributed drug information system that can be used to track the flow and consumption of antiretroviral drugs, as well as monitor how patients respond to treatment (Michael et al., 2009). The project, supported with financing, hardware, and software by Microsoft Research, is a collaborative effort of New York University's Computer Science Department and School of Medicine and the West Africa AIDS Foundation in Ghana (Microsoft Corporation, 2008).

---

aged member states "to establish or strengthen and maintain . . . health personnel information systems . . . to collect, analyze and translate data into effective health workforce policies and planning" (WHO, 2010d, p. 6). The African health workforce needs to be planned on the basis of projected needs (IOM, 2005c). Such planning must be done jointly, involving not only ministries of health but also ministries of education, finance, public service, and labor. Additionally, the private sector and the academic and medical communities should be brought to the table.

Begun in 2002 as a project to track the supply and deployment of Kenya's nursing workforce, the Kenya Health Workforce Information System (KHWIS) is today a comprehensive health workforce surveillance system that provides regulatory and staffing data on Kenya's nurses, doctors, dentists, midwives, clinical officers, and laboratory technicians and technologists. The project represents an ongoing collaboration among the Government of Kenya's Ministry of Medical Services; the Ministry of Public Health and Sanitation; and the professional nursing, medical, laboratory, and clinical officer councils. The Lillian Carter

Center for International Nursing at Emory University and the U.S. Centers for Disease Control and Prevention (CDC) provide ongoing technical assistance (Kenya Health Workforce Information System, 2010). A promising example of building African capacity for analytic planning of the health workforce, the project created a database, installed computer and satellite equipment, and trained data entry personnel on a computerized system that includes every Kenyan nurse licensed from 1960 to the present. For such efforts to be useful, they must be supported by trained statistical staff who can focus on such issues as assessment of data quality; accommodation of missing data; and estimation of temporal, geographic, and demographic trends. Developing information systems requires not just collecting data, but also sufficiently training staff in the use of systems and data analysis.

KHWIS installed hardware at the Ministry of Health offices in Nairobi and at the provincial level to facilitate the collection of deployment data. The nursing supply and regulatory database was linked with the health facility and deployment database at the Department of Nursing in the Ministry of Medical Services in Nairobi, allowing the chief nursing officer to access information on nursing workforce supply and demand. The system provides for national coordination of data collection for the entire nursing profession, a capability lacking even in industrialized countries such as the United States and the United Kingdom (Nursing Sector Study Corporation, 2004); the availability of this information provides an evidence base for decision makers on human resources for health (Riley et al., 2007). In 2009, the project was extended to other health professional cadres; it is now creating regulatory databases to track the supply of physicians, dentists, laboratory workers, and clinical officers in Kenya (Emory University School of Nursing, 2010).

Using data from the KHWIS, the Government of Kenya supported studies aimed at evaluating the country's health worker training capacity, the outcome of public–private partnerships with respect to the distribution of nurses and the subsequent effect on health services, and the impact of outmigration on Kenya's nursing workforce. Officials in Kenya's health ministry have also used information from the KHWIS to determine facility placements for newly hired personnel and identify staff qualifying for promotion, as well as employees needing to upgrade their skills (Kenya Health Workforce Information System, 2010).

Investment in women as health workers Investing in the training and education of women as health workers can have both direct and indirect positive impacts on HIV/AIDS. The direct impact is that of building the health workforce for enhanced service provision to those living with HIV/AIDS. The indirect impact is the positive downstream effect on both the health of the women themselves (a significant benefit given that women account for nearly 60 percent of HIV infections in Africa [UNAIDS, 2008]) and the health of their families and communities. Educational achievements of women can have ripple effects within the family and across generations (Belhadj and Touré, 2008) because educated women can recognize the importance of health care and know how to seek it for themselves and their children (UNFPA, 2005).

Employing women in the health workforce and thereby providing them with income has further downstream benefits. Increasing women's income has a positive impact on the educational and nutritional status of their children (Littlefield et al., 2003; Rogers and Youssef, 1988). Similarly, women's unmet contraceptive needs have been shown to decrease significantly with educational level and paid employment (Al Riyami et al., 2004). The ability to earn a decent income empowers poor women in many aspects of their lives, influencing sexual and reproductive health choices, education, and healthy behavior (UNFPA, 2007).

Utilization of the Capacity of Local Institutions

Existing local African institutions hold great potential for mitigating the future impact of the HIV/AIDS burden. The capacity of these local resources—including South–South partnerships and regional collaborations, African science academies, national public health institutes, and health resource partner institutions—should be recognized and exploited.

South–South partnerships and regional collaborations with universities and other training programs South–South partnerships and regional collaborations can be a highly effective model for diffusing successful practices. Natural partners for such collaborations include universities; public health, nursing, and medical schools; technical and vocational institutions (which serve as major sources of education and training for ancillary health workers, including the array of technicians who form the backbone of any health care system, such as laboratory technicians, X-ray technicians, and procurement specialists); and other academic training programs. Chapter 4 addresses the role of technical/vocational schools and universities in creating the health workforce of the future.

An example of a South–South partnership is a model developed by Partners in Health to build human capacity for HIV/AIDS and primary health care services in Haiti and Lesotho. Because these two countries face similar human resources challenges, they are well suited to collaboration (Ivers et al., 2010). The partnership emphasizes providing community-based support to people living with HIV/ AIDS and other diseases, recruiting and training paid community health workers in each country, developing human capacity, and scaling up services in collaboration with ministries of health (Ivers et al., 2010).

Another example of a South–South partnership is the Leadership Initiative for Public Health in East Africa (LIPHEA). LIPHEA recognizes that the health workforce in the developing world is unable to meet current health challenges, especially in the area of public health leadership. The initiative aims to strengthen the capacity of Uganda's Makerere University School of Public Health

(MUPH) and Tanzania's Muhimbili University College of Health Sciences to provide training for public health leaders, not just in Uganda and Tanzania but throughout east Africa. The goal is to establish long-term partnerships between academic institutions in the United States and east Africa and to provide substantial assistance to east Africa through curriculum revision; the development of in-service, short-term training for public health practitioners; the development of faculty who can prepare the next generation of public health professionals for national and regional public health systems; and reduction of the "brain drain" by improving professional development opportunities for public health leaders (LIPHEA, 2010).

A number of unique challenges must be overcome in creating South–South partnerships in Africa. One of these challenges is that Africans from different countries may have difficulty working together for several reasons: (1) partners from the same continent may still have cultural differences, (2) the lack of human and institutional resources is often a greater challenge for a South than for a North (developed-country) assisting partner, and (3) engaging the U.S. government team in the country in which the assisting partner is located is often challenging when the recipient partner is in a different country, because the U.S. government team does not see the benefit to its country program (Conviser, 2009). In addition, the "stovepiping" of PEPFAR funds to various African countries and to U.S. government agencies makes it difficult to undertake cooperative, multicountry projects.

African science academies Science academies, especially in resource-poor countries, are a unique resource for improving the effectiveness of a country's policies and programs involving an aspect of science, medicine, or engineering. While more economically developed countries typically have large numbers of scientists in government to call upon, the scientific capacities of less economically developed countries are more thinly spread. This situation makes it desirable to engage expertise beyond government scientists in formulating policy and implementing programs. Moreover, while scientific expertise from the international development community can be plentiful, in-country advice has particular advantages with respect to trust, contextual understanding, and sustainability (Kelley, 2009).

Unlike many sources that policy makers can tap for advice, science academies have the capability to provide balanced, multidisciplinary, authoritative, and culturally appropriate advice that is valued for its unbiased, evidence-based approach. African science academy members and those scientists appointed to academy deliberative committees tend to be the most well-known and -respected scientists and scholars in the country. As such, they are often known to the country's political leaders (Kelley, 2009). A science academy operates in a manner that is apolitical and not motivated by profit, which adds to its credibility. Likewise, most science academies receive some government funding but maintain independence from such benefactors (Hassan and Schaffer, 2009), receiving grants from private sources (Nature, 2010). African science academies can therefore offer an independent, credible perspective on politically charged issues (Hassan and Schaffer, 2009; Nature, 2010).

For example, the *HIV/AIDS, TB and Nutrition* report released in 2007 by the Academy of Science of South Africa (ASSAf) played a timely and important role in informing South African policy. ASSAf published the report when the South African Ministry of Health was taking nonscientific positions. The report was commissioned to review the scientific evidence on the dynamics of the interaction of HIV, tuberculosis (TB), and nutrition. The study panel found a dearth of data on the influence of nutrition on HIV and TB (ASSAf, 2007). The report's findings and its recommendations concerning the urgent need for research in this area were able to correct the government's prevailing misunderstandings.

Since 1986, the Institute of Medicine (IOM) has produced a series of 26 reports on various aspects of HIV/AIDS, beginning with *Confronting AIDS: Directions for Public Health, Health Care, and Research* (IOM, 1986). Other reports followed, such as *HIV and the Blood Supply: An Analysis of Crisis Decision Making*, on blood safety and HIV (IOM, 1995); *Review of the HIVNET 012 Perinatal HIV Prevention Study*, on the effectiveness of nevirapine in PMTCT (IOM, 2005b); and *Healers Abroad: Americans Responding to the Human Resource Crisis in HIV/AIDS*, addressing the crisis in human resources for health (IOM, 2005a). These reports demonstrate the range of questions that a science academy can usefully address.

The committee sees promise in the African science academies' emerging role in science and health policy at the country level, although there is much work to be done before they can become strong, self-sufficient institutions. In contrast to the high visibility of the U.S. National Academies, science academies in Africa tend to be less well funded, less active, less visible, and fewer in number (Nature, 2006). To address this problem and assist in building the capacity of African science academies, the U.S. National Academy of Sciences launched the African Science Academy Development Initiative (ASADI) (Hassan and Schaffer, 2009). ASADI's vision is to develop the capacity of African science academies so they will be regarded as trusted, credible sources of scientific advice in their respective countries (ASADI, 2008). African science academies can help bridge the gaps among technology, information, and health impact in Africa, and as they continue to evolve, their positive impacts will continue to grow.

National public health institutes National public health institutes (NPHIs) are science-based governmental organizations, such as CDC in the United States, FIOCRUZ (Fundação Oswaldo Cruz) in Brazil, RIVM (National Institute for Public Health and the Environment) in the Netherlands, and CDC in China, that provide expertise and leadership for core public health functions, including research, disease surveillance, outbreak investigation, laboratory science, policy formulation, and health education and promotion. NPHIs vary in scope, function, and size, ranging from fledgling institutes to organizations with comprehensive responsibility for research, programs, and policy for almost all public health threats. Most NPHIs, including the U.S. CDC, began as focused public health or research institutes charged with identifying and combating infectious disease threats. Over time, CDC and many other NPHIs in mid- to higher-resource countries have evolved and expanded to meet new public health challenges, including death and disability from chronic diseases, environmental and occupational threats, and injury prevention. The growth of NPHIs over the years—including both their successes and failures—provides an important frame of reference for those contexts with more limited current capacity in considering how to move forward (IANPHI, 2010; IOM, 2009).

Coordinating core public health functions through NPHIs can result in more efficient use of resources, improved delivery of public health services, and increased capacity to respond decisively to public health threats and opportunities. NPHIs are particularly beneficial in low-resource countries, where they provide public health professionals with a group of technically oriented colleagues and a prestigious career path, helping to stem the tide of experts leaving government service for higher-paying jobs with international nongovernmental organizations. NPHIs in low-resource countries also encourage governments to set science-based public health priorities and policies, better integrate and leverage funds from numerous vertical programs, and plan strategically and systematically for future human resource and infrastructure needs (IANPHI, 2010; IOM, 2009).

Moving NPHIs toward more technical depth and comprehensive capacity is the primary goal of the International Association of National Public Health Institutes (IANPHI). IANPHI serves as a professional organization for NPHI directors, assisting them in their professional and institutional growth through scientific meetings, leadership development activities, and seed grants for research and training. IANPHI's fundamental philosophy is that the collective history, knowledge, and scientific expertise of its member institutes is a powerful force for transforming public health systems in low-resource countries (IANPHI, 2010; IOM, 2009).

IANPHI is collaborating with nine low-resource countries to create new NPHIs or substantially increase capacity at fledgling institutes. Its nine long-term NPHI development sites include Burkina Faso, Ethiopia, Guinea Bissau, Mozambique, and Tanzania, with projects being explored in Bangladesh, Cambodia, Central America, and Ghana. In addition to its strategic investments of up to $670,000 in each of the nine long-term project sites, IANPHI leverages substantial strategic planning and organizational design expertise, scientific technical assistance, and public health training for each project from other IANPHI members. For example, Guinea Bissau received technical assistance and training from Brazil; Finland is providing technical assistance and training to Tanzania; the Netherlands and Norway have committed to providing assistance to Ethiopia; and Morocco has pledged technical assistance and training to Burkina Faso. In addition, IANPHI links each project with the specialized expertise of other partners, including WHO, and with key funders and programs, including the Health Metrics Network, the Global Fund, bilateral aid groups, and the U.S. government (IANPHI, 2010; IOM, 2009).

Health resource partner institutions in countries and regional networks The health and HIV/AIDS operating environment in countries (and globally) is complex and challenging. Ensuring country leadership and stewardship of the African continental response to HIV/AIDS requires the support of institutions in other countries to ensure that the HIV/AIDS agenda is permanently visible and that needed resources are mobilized both internally and externally and properly utilized. Examples of such institutions include advocacy groups, universities, science academies, professional associations, think tanks, businesses, and media. Governments are encouraged to work closely with these health resource partner institutions to strengthen national health systems for advocacy and oversight of HIV/AIDS programs, as well as the programs' integration into broader health and national development plans. At the regional level, networks of such groups already exist. For example, Equinet supports country networks of community-based health care providers, while the African Health Systems Governance Network, created in 2009 and based at the African Center for Global Health and Social Transformation (ACHEST), supports a regional network of institutions that promote better stewardship and governance of health in Africa.

Another example of a regional network is the WHO global network of collaborating centers in nursing and midwifery, whose primary responsibility is to support the regional WHO offices and the headquarters office in Geneva in achieving the MDGs. In addition to working as individual units, the centers are encouraged to maximize opportunities by working together as a network (Parfitt, 2010). More than 40 centers worldwide work in the following areas:

- Capacity building—For example, the WHO African Regional Office provided support to the University of South Africa in publishing the first African journal for nursing and midwifery researchers in the region (WHO, 2001).
- Collaborative research projects—An example is a joint research project between South Korean and Thai universities in community action research (WHO, 2001).
- Interregional initiatives—The Pan American Network for Nursing and Midwifery Collaborating Centers emphasize North–South collaborations such as that between the University of Illinois in the United States and the University of Botswana (WHO, 2001).

Strategies for the United States: Supporting Partnerships and Other Capacity-Building Programs

The United States and other donor nations can support a number of strategies in an effort to strengthen health systems, develop African institutions, and build long-term capacity so Africa can move forward independently toward a sustainable and healthier future. These strategies include institutional partnerships and other capacity-building programs.

Institutional Partnerships

A variety of institutions have engaged in partnerships to combat the burden of HIV/AIDS in Africa. Examples of partnerships between the public and private sectors, faith-based organizations (FBOs), militaries, and academic institutions are described below.

Public–private partnerships PEPFAR defines a public–private partnership as a "collaborative endeavor that combines resources from the public sector with resources from the private sector to accomplish the goals of HIV/AIDS prevention, treatment and care" (PEPFAR, 2009). Such partnerships contribute to the fight against HIV/AIDS by bringing outside resources to areas of local need. They ensure sustainability of programs by enhancing the skills and capacities of local organizations; increasing the public's access to the unique expertise and core competencies of the private sector; facilitating scale-up of proven, cost-effective interventions through private-sector networks and associations; expanding the reach of interventions by accessing target populations (for instance, through workplace programs); and sharing program costs and promoting synergy in programs. Additionally, partners make in-kind contributions that otherwise would be beyond the reach of implementers (PEPFAR, 2009).

There are many examples of successes achieved by such partnerships. In 2007, for example, PEPFAR—through CDC and Becton, Dickinson and Company (BD), a leading global medical technology company with laboratory expertise—launched a 5-year public–private partnership to improve overall laboratory systems and services in African countries severely affected by HIV/AIDS and TB (CDC, 2010). The partnership's implementation strategy includes three key components developed in collaboration with ministries of health, national reference laboratories, and implementing partners:

- country-specific laboratory strengthening programs based on national laboratory strategic plans,
- fellowship programs for BD associates to work closely with implementing partners, and

- short-term technical assistance by both BD and PEPFAR partners to provide laboratory training and develop a framework to reach all levels of laboratory service.

The collaboration is greatly expanding the amount of laboratory training offered to all PEPFAR-supported countries in Africa, and is increasing the number of health care workers trained to provide quality HIV testing and improved TB diagnostics (CDC, 2010).

In Uganda, this partnership between PEPFAR and BD implements laboratory quality management training for all laboratories performing CD4 testing and is assisting in the development of a specimen referral system for the National Tuberculosis Reference Laboratory (NTRL). To support the NTRL, the partnership uses Global Positioning System/geographic information system (GPS/GIS) technology for mapping multiple laboratory sites to develop a transportation network and monitor specific improvements in the identified laboratories (CDC, 2010).

Corporate partnerships also exist to increase African capacity for prevention of HIV/AIDS. One example is the Safe Blood for Africa program in Nigeria—a partnership among the Nigerian Ministry of Health, CDC, the U.S. Agency for International Development (USAID), and ExxonMobil. Since 2003, the program has trained more than 1,000 blood service and health care staff in how to ensure a safe blood supply. With the support of ExxonMobil, the program has provided HIV test kits to hospitals in areas of Nigeria where there previously was no capacity to conduct even minimal testing (Safe Blood for Africa Foundation, 2008).

Corporate commitment to the prevention of HIV/AIDS is also evidenced by the commitment of Pfizer, Inc. and others to the Infectious Disease Institute (IDI) in Kampala, Uganda. With help from Pfizer and others, IDI has achieved the goal of building capacity in Africa for the delivery of sustainable, high-quality prevention and care for HIV/AIDS and related infectious diseases through training and research. Since 2001, IDI has trained more than 3,500 health care providers from 27 African countries, currently providing care to approximately 10,000 patients, and has helped build research capacity in the region by pairing promising new investigators with established researchers from North America and Europe through mentoring arrangements and fellowships (Pfizer Inc., 2010).

Another example of a corporate partnership supporting HIV/AIDS prevention is the African Comprehensive HIV/AIDS Partnerships (ACHAP). Founded in 2000, ACHAP is a joint effort of the Government of Botswana, the Bill & Melinda Gates Foundation, and the Merck Company Foundation/Merck & Co., Inc. The partnership supports and enhances the government of Botswana's national response to the HIV/AIDS epidemic through a comprehensive approach to prevention, treatment, care, and support (Merck Sharp & Dohme Corporation, 2010).

Faith-based organization partnerships FBOs can make unique contributions to international development because they exist in cities, villages, and even the most rural regions of low-income countries. These organizations provide 30–40 percent of health care services in low-income countries (Kawasaki and Patten, 2002). While governments and political climates change over time, moreover, communities of faith remain intact as support systems. Box 5-2 illustrates the contributions FBOs can make to the fight against HIV/AIDS.

Military partnerships As part of the U.S. Department of Defense's directive to support foreign militaries in mitigating HIV among their forces, the U.S. Military HIV Research Program (MHRP) provides assistance to militaries in Kenya, Nigeria, and Tanzania. Various activities associated with HIV prevention, treatment, and care are carried out at military sites throughout the respective countries. These activities support services to men and women in uniform and their dependents. In Nigeria and Tanzania, these services are also provided to the civilian populations surrounding the barracks and military medical facilities. With close to 80 percent of their patient populations being civilians, these military facilities are an important component of their respective national health care systems (U.S. Military HIV Research Program, 2010).

All military–military collaborations strive to support partners' military development and strengthening of local health systems. To this end, they assist in building the partners' infrastructure and capacity to provide necessary services, including behavioral interventions tailored to the risk factors faced by their forces. In all countries, programs, initiatives, and activities are managed and overseen through direct in-country cooperation between MHRP and partners' senior military leadership (U.S. Military HIV Research Program, 2010).

In Nigeria, PEPFAR supports a military partnership with the Nigerian Armed Forces to fight HIV/AIDS. In April 2006, a need for ART services was identified in the state of Benue, which has Nigeria's highest HIV prevalence rate. With support from PEPFAR, Nigerian military staff worked in partnership with the U.S. government and key stakeholders to rapidly establish and scale up treatment services in the state (PEPFAR, 2007). A team of three Nigerian military medical staff was dispatched to assist in establishing the services. They met extensively with local support groups to ensure that the planned services would meet local needs. In June 2006, free ART was launched at the Nigerian Air Force Hospital in Makurdi, the capital of Benue. Both the Minister of State for Defense and the Governor of Benue lent political support to the inaugural program (PEPFAR, 2007).

Academic twinning The twinning relationship must exist as a partnership with parity; new skills, processes, and knowledge should be exchanged by both partners through the process (AIHA, 2005; Einterz et al., 2007). The committee

---

BOX 5-2
AIDSRelief: A Faith-Based Program
Combating HIV/AIDS in South Africa

In South Africa, the Catholic Church has provided health care in areas of need since 1849. Today there are 2 hospitals, 31 clinics, 16 hospices, 10 multipurpose health centers, numerous home-based care organizations, and hundreds of HIV projects across the Catholic dioceses in South Africa (Stark, 2010). In 2000, an AIDS Office was established to coordinate the Church's response to HIV; in 2004, the AIDS Office received PEPFAR funding through Catholic Relief Services (CRS) to provide ART and other HIV care and support services in 20 of the programs offered through the dioceses. The 5-year funding award was managed globally by CRS headquarters; the funds flowed from U.S. government channels through CRS to the implementing partners. The PEPFAR funding to CRS for ART was implemented through two local umbrella church organizations—the Institute for Youth Development South Africa (IYDSA) and the Southern African Catholic Bishops Conference (SACBC)—and became known as the AIDSRelief program. Through these programs, 73,293 people received HIV care and 35,038 were enrolled in ART over the course of 5 years (2004–2009) (Stark, 2010; Stark et al., 2010).

Beginning in 2004, AIDSRelief worked in collaboration with IYDSA and SACBC to provide community-based care and clinical treatment to people affected by HIV. Treatment facilities were expanded and equipped. Financial compliance systems were instituted, and treatment sites were prepared to implement a new electronic database to assist with patient management. Throughout the project, hundreds of health workers were trained—296 in the 2008–2009 grant year alone (Stark et al., 2010). AIDSRelief committed to supporting activities that would ensure the sustainability of treatment for people living with HIV/AIDS when donor funds were no longer available. Linkages were established with local clinical experts, as well as with health training institutions and organizations. Relationships with South African government health and social services agencies were strengthened (Stark, 2010; Stark et al., 2010).

Sustainability plans for some programs involved a variety of public–private partnership arrangements whereby government would cover the costs of certain services, including laboratory services, antiretroviral drugs, and even staff salaries. For other programs, sustaining people on ART involved the transfer of patients to South African government health services as they became available and accessible. Over the 5 years, 6,764 patients have been transferred to accredited government facilities where they will continue to receive lifelong treatment. The strong partnership with the local church, the commitment to collaborate with the local government, and the encouragement and support of the activity manager at the U.S. government mission in South Africa made the transfers possible (Stark, 2010; Stark et al., 2010).

The program is currently embarking on a new direction, with local South African organizations taking the lead. The local organizations now receive their PEPFAR grant funds directly from the U.S. government and are responsible for managing all aspects of the program. AIDSRelief will serve its partners as a subgrantee in specified technical areas and will support partners as they assume their new role. South Africa's is the first of the PEPFAR HIV/AIDS treatment programs to transition to local leadership (Stark, 2010; Stark et al., 2010).

believes that parity is both a necessary and defining characteristic of a twinning relationship.

Formed in 1992, the **American International Health Alliance (AIHA)**[7] broke ground for the establishment of large-scale twinning relationships aimed at building sustainable institutional and human resource capacity in nations with limited resources. AIHA was initially established by a consortium of major health care provider associations and professional medical education organizations to help the nations of the former Soviet Union build much-needed health system capacity (AIHA, 2010a). In 2004, AIHA established the HIV/AIDS Twinning Center, which creates peer-to-peer relationships between organizations working to improve services for people living with or affected by HIV/AIDS; the Twinning Center currently has programs in 11 countries in Africa and continues its program in Russia (AIHA, 2007).

An example of university twinning is the **Academic Model for Providing Access to Healthcare (AMPATH)**, a partnership among Moi University School of Medicine, Moi Teaching and Referral Hospital, and other health centers and hospitals operated by Kenya's Ministry of Health and a consortium of North American institutions led by Indiana University.[8] AMPATH aims to deliver essential primary care services, control HIV/AIDS, and mitigate its economic and social consequences in a population of 2 million people in western Kenya (Einterz et al., 2007, 2010; Kimaiyo, 2010). In contrast with most academic twinning HIV/AIDS care programs, which partner with the private sector, delivery of care through AMPATH occurs through the public sector (Einterz et al., 2010; Kimaiyo, 2010).

AMPATH is supported by more than 1,000 staff members: 42 staff from Moi University; 447 staff from the Kenyan Ministry of Health; 665 direct AMPATH employees; and 8 North Americans (Kimaiyo, 2010), at least one of whom is an Indiana University general internal medicine faculty member committed on-site in Kenya (Einterz et al., 2007). In addition to care provided for patients, Indiana University School of Medicine helps educate and train Kenyan physicians in clinical care and research through a partnership called ASANTE (America/

---

[7] AIHA operates under various cooperative agreements and grants from U.S. and international donor agencies, including USAID; the U.S. Department of Health and Human Services, Health Resources and Services Administration (HRSA); WHO; the Global Fund to Fight AIDS, Tuberculosis and Malaria; and the German Society for Technical Cooperation (AIHA, 2010b).

[8] The partnership has been funded in the past by PEPFAR, CDC, the Maternal to Child Transmission Plus Initiative, the Bill & Melinda Gates Foundation, and other private philanthropic funds (Einterz et al., 2007). The consortium of North American institutions also includes Duke University, Brown University, the University of Utah, the University of Toronto, George Washington University, and Purdue University.

sub-Saharan Africa Network for Training and Education in Medicine).[9] More than 800 Kenyans and Americans have participated in exchanges of students, faculty, and postgraduates through this partnership.

AMPATH's emphasis is not on the twinning relationship between two universities but on a triadic relationship among the two universities and the ministry of health (Einterz et al., 2007, 2010). Indiana University also ensures that there is Kenyan leadership at every level of the program; thus, Moi University is fully invested and shares equal ownership of the program (Kimaiyo, 2010).

Another example of twinning is the **International Training and Education Center on Health (I-TECH)**,[10] a global network that works with local partners to develop skilled health care workers and strong national health systems in resource-limited countries, promoting local ownership to sustain effective health systems (Holmes, 2004; I-TECH, 2010). Table 5-3 summarizes I-TECH's principal programs and activities and the services they provide. The benefits of selected I-TECH programs are summarized later in the chapter.

Like AMPATH, I-TECH recognizes the importance of including local governing bodies and organizations to build a broad base of support among multiple stakeholders. I-TECH adapts each program to local preferences and resource constraints. To ensure the efficacy of each program, I-TECH invests in operations research and formal process evaluations. Ongoing monitoring allows for midstream corrections, as findings are communicated to program managers to improve decision making (I-TECH, 2009c).

Other Capacity-Building Programs

Other capacity-building programs include foundation programs and initiatives of civil society organizations.

Foundation programs Capacity-building efforts should target not only key health personnel in the health system, but also individuals in country governments who require capacity building for leadership. Governments act as stewards of the public interest and are responsible for ensuring conditions that allow their citizens to be as healthy as possible. Ministries of health and the ministers who lead them must be able to perform a set of core stewardship functions within the ministry and across the government. Ministers and ministries of health are currently

---

[9] Other North American institutions participating in ASANTE include Brown Medical School, Duke University School of Medicine, Lehigh Valley Hospital and Health Network, Providence Portland Medical Center, the University of Utah School of Medicine, and the University of Toronto Faculty of Medicine.

[10] I-TECH serves many countries in Africa, including Botswana, Ethiopia, Kenya, Malawi, Mozambique, Namibia, Tanzania, South Africa, and Uganda. It receives funding from HRSA, USAID, the U.S. CDC, and the U.S. Department of Defense. Most of I-TECH's partnerships, however, are sponsored by PEPFAR (I-TECH, 2009c).

TABLE 5-3 I-TECH's Principal Programs

Program	Activities	Services Provided
Health System Strengthening	Strengthening of clinical care and treatment systems	• I-TECH clinical mentors who help partners develop goals and test new methods of care • Quality improvement programs to strengthen systems of care
	Strengthening of health information systems	• Electronic medical record systems • Training management systems • Remote clinical diagnostic systems
	Strengthening of laboratory systems	• Up-to-date materials and supplies • Laboratory information systems • Training and support for new diagnostics
	Strengthening of training and education systems	• Services to strengthen educational institutions that coordinate, design, deliver, monitor, and evaluate courses, degree programs, and workshops on infectious diseases
Health Workforce Development	Health care worker education systems	• Collaborative programs with the ministry of health and ministry of education • Reform of educational degree programs • Integration of evidence-based information on infectious diseases into existing courses • Faculty development training
	Training development	• Interactive training for diverse cadres of health care providers and educators • Multimedia resources
	Distance learning	• Distance learning for environments with limited technology and low bandwidth • Learning opportunities that allow students to remain on the job
	Clinical mentoring	• A venue for health care workers to practice hands-on skills with oversight by an experienced provider
Operations Research and Evaluation	Monitoring and evaluation	• Research designs and methods for resource-limited settings • Operations research to inform every phase of programming, starting with assessments before an intervention begins

TABLE 5-3 Continued

Program	Activities	Services Provided
Prevention, Care, and Treatment of Infectious Diseases	Prevention	• Training of health care workers in infection control • Behavior change communication interventions • Prevention with HIV-positive clients
	Care and treatment	• Technical assistance on clinical care

SOURCE: I-TECH, 2009c.

overlooked, however, when investments are made and initiatives are designed to strengthen health systems (Omaswa and Ivey Boufford, 2010).

The W.K. Kellogg Foundation was established in 1930 with the purpose of administering funds to promote the welfare, health, education, and safeguarding of children and youth. Over the years, the foundation's programming has continued to evolve, striving to remain innovative and responsive to the ever-changing needs of society (W.K. Kellogg Foundation, 2010a). In 1989, the Kellogg International Leadership Program (KILP) was formed to promote the development of leadership capacity by connecting leaders in Latin America, the Caribbean, the United States, and Southern Africa. Through seminars, small study groups, and community-focused projects, KILP fellows obtain both didactic training and hands-on experience to refine their global leadership skills. Priority is given to leaders in the sectors most aligned with Kellogg's four levers of change: civic responsibility, economic opportunity, skills and leadership, and health and well-being (W.K. Kellogg Foundation, 2010b).

Dr. Sheila Tlou, now UNAIDS Regional Support Team Director for East and Southern Africa (September 2010) and a former Minister of Health of Botswana (2004–2009), was the first recipient of the KILP grant. With the grant, she received her Ph.D. in the United States in community health nursing, with a concentration in gender and health issues, and she is now vice chair of a coalition of 20 women's organizations that focus on issues of women's political, health, and economic empowerment; violence; human rights; and education of girls. In addition, Tlou cofounded the Coping Centre for People Living with AIDS in Gabarone, Botswana, which rehabilitates HIV-positive women and develops their capacity to be leaders in the community. As a researcher, Tlou was instrumental in convincing Botswana's government to invest in home care and treatment for HIV/AIDS patients. She served as HIV coordinator for the University of Botswana and is a highly regarded voice in the community, civic, and government sectors. Tlou is one of many successful public health and government leaders developed through this grant program (W.K. Kellogg Foundation, 2010b).

Additional government capacity-building programs include the Humphrey Fellowship Program and the Fogarty Fellowship Program. Sponsored by the U.S. Department of State, the Humphrey Fellowship Program provides midcareer professionals from developing countries with 10 months of nondegree academic study and professional enrichment in the United States (Hubert H. Humphrey Fellowship Program, 2007). The program offers fellows valuable opportunities for leadership development and professional engagement. More than 3,700 men and women have been honored as Humphrey Fellows since the program began in 1978 (Hubert H. Humphrey Fellowship Program, 2007). The Fogarty Fellowship Program promotes productive reentry of National Institutes of Health (NIH)–trained foreign investigators into their home countries upon completion of their experiences with the fellowship program (NIH, 2010).

Civil society organization initiatives Throughout history, civil society organizations have been known to contribute to the good of the world. In keeping with this historical role, Rotary International formed Rotarians For Fighting AIDS, Inc. (RFFA) in 2003. RFFA's mission is to improve the lives of orphans and vulnerable children affected by HIV/AIDS by mobilizing Rotarians and partners to provide care, nutrition, education, and life skills (RFFA, 2010a). RFFA works closely with the African Network for Children Orphaned and at Risk (ANCHOR), a partnership among four entities: RFFA, Project HOPE (Health Opportunities for People Everywhere), the Coca-Cola Africa Foundation, and Emory University's School of Public Health (RFFA, 2010b).

RFFA's current initiatives are focused on addressing issues related to HIV/AIDS orphans and vulnerable children. Through projects such as Orphan Rescue, RFFA has partnered with ANCHOR to build the capacity of families and local communities to cope with and respond to the needs of these children. The project provides vital educational support in the form of nutrition, uniforms, supplies, and mandatory school fees (RFFA, 2010c).

Another noteworthy project creates Kidz Clubs—community meeting places that provide children safe spaces to meet, play, and interact. RFFA and ANCHOR have successfully assisted communities in developing more than 250 Kidz Clubs across seven African countries, reaching and caring for more than 20,000 needy children affected by HIV/AIDS. In these clubs, children learn coping skills and build resilience. Counseling is provided to children dealing with grief, loss, violence, and other challenges resulting from HIV/AIDS (RFFA, 2010b).

Benefits of Partnerships and Other Capacity-Building Programs

As evidenced by the preceding examples of partnerships and training programs, many benefits are realized by participants. Among these benefits are increased program effectiveness and the opportunity to network and participate in the global health movement.

Increased program effectiveness The accomplishments of I-TECH's HIV/ART Nurse Specialist (HANS) Training Program illustrate the benefits of capacity-building initiatives. As a result of this program, for example, the number of Ethiopian nurse mentors who were once themselves HANS trainees has increased over time. This outcome reflects the expanded role of nurses as a result of the program, and indicates the program's success in achieving the goal of building capacity within the Ethiopian health care system to train the nursing workforce in HIV/AIDS specialist care (I-TECH, 2009b). Participants' pre- and posttests showed a significant increase in knowledge. More important, participants demonstrated consistent improvement in the performance of key competencies during their clinical practicum (I-TECH, 2009b).

Likewise, I-TECH's *Program Evaluation for the Implementation of the Revised Syndromic Management Algorithms for Sexually Transmitted Infections in Two Districts in Botswana* found that, relative to patients at comparison clinics, a higher percentage of patients of trainees reported that the provider (1) offered an HIV test (87 percent versus 29 percent), (2) conducted a physical examination (98 percent versus 64 percent), (3) helped them develop a plan to avoid future acquisition of sexually transmitted infections (STIs) (95 percent versus 76 percent), and (4) provided patient-specific information about HIV risk (65 percent versus 32 percent) (I-TECH, 2009d; Weaver et al., 2008).

As a final example, at IDI in Uganda, a 4-week course on comprehensive management of HIV/AIDS, including ART, improved the clinical skills of doctors in 11 of 17 areas evaluated. Interactive methods, such as hands-on practice sessions, case discussions, and role-play, were effective in changing physician practices and in some cases the health outcomes of patients (I-TECH, 2009a; Weaver et al., 2006).

Opportunity to network and participate in the global health movement Twinning and partnering can contribute to greater networking by exposing partners to each other's existing networks (ICAD, 1999). An unprecedented enthusiasm for global health currently exists among students and medical residents in U.S. universities (Drain et al., 2007; IOM, 2009). In 2008, the Consortium of Universities on Global Health created a formal alliance to build collaborations and foster the exchange of knowledge and experience among interdisciplinary university global health programs, working across education, research, and service (CUGH, 2010). The private sector and professional associations also have demonstrated an interest in sharing their business and technical acumen for the greater social good (IOM, 2009). In this context, participating in an international twinning relationship or partnership is beneficial to the Northern partner in that such programs attract faculty, students, and employees at the respective universities or organizations. Further, academic institutions are much more likely to be successful in both launching and sustaining global health programs if they work with international partners (Koplan and Baggett, 2008).

Challenges of Partnerships and Other Capacity-Building Programs

Although capacity-building programs have achieved many successes, they have faced challenges as well. Evaluations of twinning and other capacity-building programs reveal the following challenges to the future success or replication of such programs.

Financing WHO estimated that it would cost $254.8 billion in training and recurrent salary costs over 10 years to eliminate the global human resource gap (of 4.3 million health workers) (WHO, 2006). The question immediately arises of whether and how governments in low-income countries can finance such scale-up of human resources. Already, human resource spending can consume more than half of ministries' recurrent health expenditures (WHO, 2008b). Expanded numbers of health workers require expanded resources to pay the costs of their employment, including wages and benefits, as well as the cost of their education and training, including teacher salaries; books, laboratories, and equipment; new buildings, classrooms, offices, and laboratories; maintenance and repair of facilities and equipment; and students' living expenses. Scaling up of the health workforce also requires simultaneous increases in other health goods, such as drugs, supplies, functioning equipment, and adequate management and supervision (WHO, 2008b).

Given the extent of these costs, external support may be necessary to supplement domestic resources in scaling up the health workforce. To ensure the long-term sustainability of such a scale-up, donors must work within each country's strategic plan, and a maximum amount of domestic resources must be mobilized. It has been noted that donors have been reluctant in the past to fund recurrent costs, such as employment costs of health workers (Vujicic, 2005), although some donors, such as the Global Fund, reportedly have begun to be more flexible in their policies concerning financing of public-sector recurrent costs (WHO, 2008b). The effect of external assistance on the ability of countries to scale up the health workforce is likely to be small, however; even a doubling of external assistance would not be as powerful as the combination of substantial economic growth and governments allocating larger shares of their spending to health (Preker et al., 2007). Ultimately, then, countries need to make choices about the scale-up of their health workforce that best suit their epidemiological profile and fiscal circumstances (WHO, 2008b).

Sustainability Sustaining twinning projects or other partnerships over time may be challenging, often because of insufficient funding and high administrative costs (ICAD, 1999). As noted earlier, for example, the AMPATH twin in Kenya maintains a staff that includes 665 direct employees and 8 North Americans (Kimaiyo, 2010), at least one of whom is an Indiana University general internal medicine faculty member committed on-site in Kenya (Einterz et al., 2007). The cost of maintaining such numbers of staff may be prohibitive in some settings. In addition, stagnant funding is increasing the burden on the program to expand services while working with fewer resources (USAID-AMPATH, 2010).

More pressing priorities Some organizations involved in twinning or other partnership or training programs may need to devote all of their energies to the survival of their regular programs (ICAD, 1999). This pressure is bilateral; both partners have pressing priorities beyond the twinning project or partnership. In some countries, a program may not be seen as contributing to PEPFAR goals. Those goals call for reaching large numbers of people with services; some 85 percent of U.S. funds going to Africa have been for PEPFAR, so this is a high priority for U.S. missions in the region. Twinning projects are thought to contribute relatively little to the achievement of PEPFAR's goals, and it is not always clear at the outset how such projects may fit into broader country plans. Hence it has sometimes been difficult to obtain buy-in for projects in Africa for which twinning would be appropriate, and some of the earliest twinning projects in the region could not fit readily into the existing programs of U.S. government teams (Conviser, 2009).

Time frame of results Relative to one-shot technical assistance programs, twinning programs take time to establish because they depend on the development of institutional and interpersonal relationships. Also, twinning programs require about the same amount of administrative oversight from in-country U.S. government agencies as larger-budget PEPFAR programs and may be slower to produce results. In-country U.S. government teams have often felt it was not worth the effort to fund relatively small projects that require roughly the same amount of attention as far larger PEPFAR initiatives (Conviser, 2009).

Lack of appropriate infrastructure Most African organizations lack an established infrastructure equipped to serve twinning or training projects (ICAD, 1999), and many of those evaluated have noted information technology challenges (Kangas et al., 2010). Several twinning projects (including projects in Botswana, Zambia, and Ethiopia) have reported that technology was a challenge in maintaining the twinning relationship. Fragile e-mail systems made it difficult to exchange information between partners. Limited access to electricity and telephone landlines was also cited as hampering communication between partners (Conviser, 2009). The AMPATH partnership in Kenya reported difficulties in encouraging patients' continued compliance with ART (with a rate of loss to follow-up of 1.6 percent in the first quarter of 2010) as a result of several constraints, including limited access to program vehicles, a lack of reliable public transportation for both outreach staff and patients, and inadequacy of the electronic tracking system in locating patients. Some health care facilities lacked supplies needed to provide STI care, such as patient education materials, condoms, and contact slips (I-TECH, 2009d; Weaver et al., 2008).

Extra strain on overburdened staff In low-resource countries, the human resource crisis leaves hospital staff members extremely busy, limiting their communication with twinning partners between visits. The amount of administrative work required for the relatively small-scale twinning projects does not differ significantly from the amount of work necessary for much larger projects, challenging small and already overburdened staff (Conviser, 2009). AMPATH's outreach and follow-up with current patients, for example, were challenged by a shortage of staffing, as reported in the quarterly PEPFAR performance review for January–March 2010 (USAID-AMPATH, 2010).

Lack of an in-country coordinator The AIHA HIV/AIDS Twinning Center's evaluation described one challenge particular to that organization. The absence of U.S. Health Resources and Services Administration (HRSA) representatives from U.S. government teams or an AIHA office in Africa makes it more administratively complex for other U.S. government agencies to fund twinning projects: U.S. government agencies must designate the funds for HRSA, which passes them on to AIHA, which provides them to the partners. The funding agencies also must do a substantial amount of administrative work on these small-ticket projects, whose impact in meeting PEPFAR goals, as noted above, may be both minor and delayed. There needs to be a single point of contact for both HRSA and the organization serving as its agent in overseeing twinning projects in Africa, with regular scheduled communication between them. This would help promote both advocacy and accountability in twinning projects, although it would come at the cost of increased work for HRSA's agent(s) in Africa (Conviser, 2009).

RECOMMENDATIONS

Recommendation 5-1: *Analyze and plan for meeting workforce requirements.* African governments and international organizations should assess and plan for meeting national workforce requirements for responding to the long-term burden of HIV/AIDS.

- **Recommendation 5-1a:** Through partnership programs and other investments, African governments and institutions, along with U.S. private companies, academic institutions, foundations, and civil society organizations, should establish national databases and information systems for health care worker statistics, as well as bolster the analytic capacity of national planners for determining human resource needs.
- **Recommendation 5-1b:** African governments and institutions should create staffing models to optimize the impact of the health care work-

force. Such models should include developing cadres of managers and support staff outside the clinical health sector, encouraging needs-based training and task sharing within the health sector, focusing on retention through compensation and other incentives, utilizing information technologies, and harnessing the informal health sector.

- **Recommendation 5-1c:** In Africa, governments and institutions should work together in planning the African health care workforce based on projected needs derived from national data and analyses of future human resource requirements. Such planning should involve ministries of health, education, finance, public service, and labor. The private sector and the academic and medical communities should also be brought to the table for such national human resource planning exercises.

Recommendation 5-2: *Utilize existing African capacity.* African governments and international donors should recognize, invest in, strengthen, and utilize currently existing capacity within African institutions and networks to provide local solutions for responding to the HIV/AIDS epidemic. This capacity includes South–South and regional partnerships, universities, African science academies, national public health institutes, and other networks within Africa.

Recommendation 5-3: *Develop government leadership and management in health.* U.S. government agencies and programs, foundations, and academic institutions should invest in the development of African leadership and management in the health sector.

- **Recommendation 5-3a:** U.S. government agencies, such as the Health Resources and Service Administration (HRSA), the U.S. Agency for International Development (USAID), and the U.S. Centers for Disease Control and Prevention (CDC) and its global counterparts, should be actively engaged in leadership and management development, and the International Association of Public Health Institutes should be tapped as a resource for advancing these efforts.
- **Recommendation 5-3b:** U.S. foundations and academic institutions should invest in African leadership and management development through programs that educate African scientists and scholars who may then take on leadership positions in their own countries.

Recommendation 5-4: *Invest in innovative partnerships.* Private-sector organizations, professional organizations, faith-based organizations, academic and research institutions, militaries, foundations, and civil society organizations should increase funding for and participation in meaningful, effective, and innovative partnerships designed to build African capacity now to address the full extent of the HIV/AIDS burden over the next 10 years.

- **Recommendation 5-4a:** New U.S.–African partnerships between local vocational or technical schools that train allied health professionals, laboratory technicians, informatics specialists, and/or health administrators should be explored and encouraged.
- **Recommendation 5-4b:** Innovative North–South and South–South partnerships that build human resources for health should be developed. In North–South partnerships, African counterparts should take the lead in developing and controlling the partnership agenda.

As a final note, the committee emphasizes that a formidable gap exists between innovations in health (including vaccines, drugs, and strategies for care) and their delivery to communities in the developing world (Madon et al., 2007). Many of the recommendations in this chapter imply a need to perform operations research[11] (OR) and implementation research[12] (IR)—as well as ongoing evaluation—of programs, partnerships, and interventions aimed at combating HIV/AIDS in Africa. Such efforts can identify the optimal and most efficient approaches for carrying out the committee's recommendations. Because HIV/AIDS is a mosaic of epidemics in Africa (see Chapter 1), programs and policies will require tailoring to local circumstances. There is a wide range of OR opportunities in capacity building for HIV/AIDS, including identifying the best methods for:

- obtaining and delivering commodities in the health system;
- making mass treatment more feasible;
- managing patients on fewer doses of ART;
- treating for a period of time and then stopping treatment, but monitoring the patient;
- preventing infections and changing behavior in a particular context or risk group;
- using new communication tools and social media to reach those in need of prevention messages;
- scaling up information and communication technology;
- employing task/responsibility sharing;
- packaging together interventions for HIV/AIDS, TB, and other diseases;

---

[11] Operations research seeks to identify and address barriers related to the performance of specific projects (Madon et al., 2007).

[12] Implementation research seeks to create generalizable knowledge that can be applied across settings and contexts to answer central questions (such as how multiple interventions can be packaged effectively to capture cost efficiencies and to reduce the splintering of health systems into disease-specific programs) (Madon et al., 2007).

- training a new generation of researchers to bridge the implementation gap; and
- strengthening research institutions in low-income countries (Madon et al., 2007).

The recommendations in this chapter, therefore, should be tested, evaluated, and tailored to specific country and regional contexts.

REFERENCES

Accordia Global Health Foundation. 2010. *Return on investment: The long-term impact of building healthcare capacity in Africa.* Washington, DC: Accordia Global Health Foundation.

AIHA (American International Health Alliance). 2005. *HIV/AIDS twinning center frequently asked questions.* http://www.twinningagainstaids.org/faq.html (accessed November 2, 2009).

———. 2007. *HIV/AIDS twinning center: Overview.* http://www.twinningagainstaids.org/overview.html (accessed August 16, 2010).

———. 2010a. *History.* http://www.aiha.com/en/WhoWeAre/History.asp (accessed August 12, 2010).

———. 2010b. *Who we are.* http://www.aiha.com/en/WhoweAre/ (accessed August 12, 2010).

Al Riyami, A., M. Afifi, and R. M. Mabry. 2004. Women's autonomy, education and employment in Oman and their influence on contraceptive use. *Reproductive Health Matters* 12(23):144-154.

AMREF (African Medical and Research Foundation). 2010. *Traditional healers, South Africa.* http://www.amref.org/what-we-do/traditional-healers-south-africa/ (accessed July 31, 2010).

ASADI (African Science Academy Development Initiative). 2008. *African science academy development intiative: Progress and promise.* http://www.nationalacademies.org/asadi/progressreport.pdf (accessed December 20, 2010).

ASSAf (Academy of Science of South Africa). 2007. *HIV, TB and nutrition: Scientific inquiry into the nutritional influences on human immunity with special reference to HIV infection and active TB in South Africa.* Pretoria, South Africa: ASSAf.

August-Brady, M. 2010. *Nursing and nursing education in Mozambique from Michele August-Brady.* http://www.nursingsociety.org/VolunteerConnect/Pages/NursingMozambique.aspx (accessed October 28, 2010).

Avert. 2010. *Why HIV and AIDS home based care?* http://www.avert.org/aids-home-care.htm (accessed July 13, 2010).

Belhadj, H., and A. Touré. 2008. Gender equality and the right to health. *The Lancet* 372(9655): 2008-2009.

Buchan, J., and M. R. Del Poz. 2003. Role definitions, skill mix, multi-skilling and "new" workers. In *Towards a global health workforce strategy*, edited by P. Ferrinho and M. R. Del Poz. Antwerp, Belgium: ITGPress. Pp. 275-300.

CDC (Centers for Disease Control and Prevention). 2010. *Public-private partnership strengthens global laboratory systems.* http://www.cdc.gov/globalaids/Success-Stories/BD-Public-Private-Partnership.html (accessed August 9, 2010).

Chen, L., T. Evans, S. Anand, J. I. Boufford, H. Brown, M. Chowdhury, M. Cueto, L. Dare, G. Dussault, G. Elzinga, E. Fee, D. Habte, P. Hanvoravongchai, M. Jacobs, C. Kurowski, S. Michael, A. Pablos-Mendez, N. Sewankambo, G. Solimano, B. Stilwell, A. de Waal, and S. Wibulpolprasert. 2004. Human resources for health: Overcoming the crisis. *The Lancet* 364(9449):1984-1990.

Commission for Africa. 2005. *Our common interest: Report of the Commission for Africa.* 2005. London: Commission for Africa.

Conviser, R. 2009. *Building capacity from within: AIHA's twinning program in Africa.* Missoula, MT: Global Health Policy Partners.

CUHG (Consortium of Universities for Global Health). 2010. *Background.* http://www.cugh.org/about/background (accessed August 23, 2010).

Dada, J., Fantsuam Foundation, V. Francis, Emerging Markets Group, M. Isaac, M. Mayson, Catholic Relief Services, T. Mensah, and Sinapi Aba Trust. 2009. *Partnership models for successful microenterprise service delivery to HIV and AIDS-affected communities.* Washington, DC: USAID.

Dare, L. 2010. *Evaluating health systems.* Presentation to the IOM committee on planning the evaluation of PEPFAR. http://www.iom.edu/~/media/Files/Activity%20Files/Global/PEPFAR2/Lola%20Dare.ashx (accessed September 22, 2010).

Dohrn, J., B. Nzama, and M. Murrman. 2009. The impact of HIV scale-up on the role of nurses in South Africa: Time for a new approach. *Journal of Acquired Immune Deficiency Syndromes* 52:S27-S29.

Dovlo, D. 2003. *The brain drain and retention of health professionals in Africa.* Paper presented at regional training conference on improving tertiary education in sub-Saharan Africa: Things that work!, Accra, Ghana, September 23-25.

Drain, P. K., A. Primack, D. D. Hunt, W. W. Fawzi, K. K. Holmes, and P. Gardner. 2007. Global health in medical education: A call for more training and opportunities. *Academic Medicine* 82(3):226-230.

Eckhert, N. L. 2002. The global pipeline: Too narrow, too wide or just right? *Medical Education* 36(7):606-613.

Einterz, R. M., S. Kimaiyo, H. N. K. Mengech, B. O. Khwa-Otsyula, F. Esamai, F. Quigley, and J. J. Mamlin. 2007. Responding to the HIV pandemic: The power of an academic medical partnership. *Academic Medicine* 82(8):812-818.

Einterz, R. M., J. Mamlin, W. Tierney, P. Biondich, D. Litzelman, M. Were, and T. Inui. 2010. *AMPATH.* Presentation to the IOM committee on envisioning a strategy to prepare for the long-term burden of HIV/AIDS: African needs and U.S. interests, Washington, DC, February 4, 2010.

eMOCHA (electronic Mobile Open-source Comprehensive Health Application). 2010. *eMOCHA: Electronic mobile open-source comprehensive health application.* http://emocha.org/ (accessed July 29, 2010).

Emory University School of Nursing. 2010. *Health workforce information systems–Kenya project.* http://www.nursing.emory.edu/lccin/research/health_workforce/project_kenya.html (accessed September 2, 2010).

Ferrinho, P., I. Fronteira, M. Sidat, F. da Sousa, and G. Dussault. 2010. Profile and professional expectations of medical students in Mozambique: A longitudinal study. *Human Resources for Health* 8(1):21.

Fox, S., C. Fawcett, K. Kelly, and P. Ntlabati. 2002. *Integrated Community-based Home Care (ICHC) in South Africa: A review of the model implemented by the Hospice Association of South Africa.* Capetown, South Africa: The Centre for AIDS Development, Research and Evaluation (Cadre) on behalf of The POLICY Project.

Glenngård, A. H., and A. Anell. 2003. *Investment in human resources for health problems, approaches and donor experiences.* Joint Learning Initiative on human resources for health and development. JLI working paper 2-6.

Hassan, M. H. A., and D. Schaffer. 2009. When less is more but still not enough: Managing academies of science in a globalised world. *International Journal of Technology Management* 46(1-2):71-82.

High-Level Forum on the Health MDGs. 2004. *Addressing Africa's health workforce crisis: An avenue for action.* Abuja, Nigeria: World Bank and WHO.

Holmes, K. 2004. *Model of training for grassroots work on HIV.* Paper read at the December 1, 2004 workshop of the IOM committee on overseas placement of U.S. healthcare professionals, Washington, DC.

———. 2010b. *Análise dos recursos humanos da saúde (RHS) nos países africanos de língua oficial portuguesa (PALOP).* Geneva: WHO.

———. 2010c. *eHealth for health care delivery.* http://www.who.int/eht/eHealthHCD/en/index.html (accessed August 5, 2010).

———. 2010d. *International recruitment of health personnel: Draft global code of practice.* Paper presented at sixty-third world health assembly, Geneva, Switzerland, May 20.

Zachariah, R., N. Ford, M. Philips, S. Lynch, M. Massaquoi, V. Janssens, and A. D. Harries. 2009. Task shifting in HIV/AIDS: Opportunities, challenges and proposed actions for sub-Saharan Africa. *Transactions of the Royal Society of Tropical Medicine and Hygiene* 103(6):549-558.

6

Strategies to Ensure Ethical Decision-Making Capacity for HIV/AIDS: Policy and Programming in Africa

---

Key Findings

- A gap exists between treatment needs and resources in Africa. Difficult questions will inevitably arise regarding how to prioritize access to treatment ethically and equitably.
- When people whose needs exceed available resources have approximately the same clinical status or risk exposure, medical criteria alone are insufficient to guide resource allocation decisions, as will often be the case with needs for HIV/AIDS prevention, treatment, and care.
- Many key decision makers in Africa need assistance in developing capacities for ethical decision making for policies, programs, and resource allocation with respect to HIV/AIDS in their populations.

If global donor resources remain constrained and the predicted burden of HIV/AIDS in Africa over the next decade ensues, difficult questions will inevitably arise regarding how to prioritize access to treatment ethically and equitably; the answers to these questions will have profound ethical implications. This chapter examines these ethical issues, focusing on options for building ethical decision-making capacity in Africa as a complement to the discussion of strategies to build capacity for prevention, treatment, and care in Chapter 5.

The long-term burden of HIV/AIDS will coexist with African health systems' many other responsibilities toward the populations they serve, including overall health system functioning, maternal and child health, prevention and treatment of infectious conditions other than HIV, injury prevention and care, mental health, and chronic conditions such as cancer and cardiovascular disease. Likewise, governments and donors have ethical obligations to address the full range of pressing global health needs, which can represent competing moral claims on limited resources. At the same time, HIV/AIDS may be exceptional in that the disease usually strikes individuals at the prime of their lives for working, having children, and supporting families. Issues of the ethical allocation of health resources between HIV/AIDS and other health needs is beyond the scope of this study. Those issues aside, however, the prevalence of HIV/AIDS is expected to increase for the forseeable future (see Chapter 2 and Appendix A). Therefore, significant resources will need to be dedicated to combating the epidemic (IOM, 2005), and this chapter addresses ethical issues regarding the utilization of those resources.

The starting point for the discussion is the expectation that needs for HIV/AIDS prevention, treatment, and care will vastly exceed the resources available to meet those needs in resource-constrained African countries where the projected long-term burden of HIV/AIDS is very high. The combination of "high prevalence, low incomes, and heavy dependence on external assistance" in many African countries is of particular concern (Project HOPE, 2009; Haacker, 2009). Within the sphere of HIV/AIDS, many competing claims on resources will continue to arise: between subpopulations of persons who need antiretroviral treatment (e.g., in some circumstances, between those requiring their first treatment regimen and those requiring second- and third-line regimens); between subpopulations of persons who need preventive interventions; and among efforts to provide ART, HIV/AIDS care, and preventive interventions (see Chapter 2 for a discussion of these trade-offs). Such trade-offs are and will continue to be a reality, and the ways in which policy makers and others weigh them and their consequences are at the heart of this ethical inquiry. Whatever the outcome of the decisions made regarding the allocation of resources in the context of HIV/AIDS in Africa, those decisions will make an enormous difference in the lives of large numbers of people living with HIV/AIDS.

This chapter first reviews existing principles for ethical decisions in health care that have been promulgated by international organizations. The subsequent section examines how an ethical decision-making capacity for HIV/AIDS policy and programming can be developed in Africa.

EXISTING PRINCIPLES FOR ETHICAL
DECISIONS IN HEALTH CARE

This section examines in turn the levels of decision making in the allocation of health resources; key moral imperatives; the concept of equal moral status; and international covenants, codes, and declarations on ethics.

Levels of Decision Making in the Allocation of Health Resources

The World Medical Association's (WMA's) *Medical Ethics Manual* identifies three levels of decision making for the allocation of health resources (Williams, 2009). Important ethical responsibilities exist at all three levels because decisions at each level are based on values and have significant consequences for the health and well-being of individuals and communities (Williams, 2009). At the *macro* level, governments determine the overall health budget and its distribution across such categories as human resources, hospital operating expenses, research, and disease-specific treatment programs (Williams, 2009). Given the projected increase in workload associated with managing the HIV/AIDS epidemic, for example, governments must make decisions at this macro level to ensure an adequate and competent workforce (see the discussion of optimizing the existing workforce in Chapter 5). Additionally, policy makers must consider competing societal goods, such as transportation, education, energy, and employment, especially since multiple socioeconomic determinants have powerful effects on the health of individuals and populations. At the *meso* level, institutions such as ministries of health, hospitals, and clinics determine which services they will provide and how much they will spend on such expenses as staff, equipment, and supplies (Williams, 2009). At the *micro* level, health care providers decide what expenditures to recommend for the benefit of each individual patient, such as tests, referrals, hospitalization, and generic versus brand-name pharmaceuticals (Williams, 2009).

Key Moral Imperatives

The committee identified two key imperatives it believes should guide ethical decision making: (1) at the macro and meso levels, to pursue justice in the distribution of benefits and burdens; and (2) at the micro level, to ensure that decisions are in the best interests of patients.

Ethical decisions at the macro and meso levels should equitably protect the interests of everyone who stands to lose or gain from those decisions. At their gravest, decisions on resource allocation can deny life-saving prevention or treatment to patients in need. A morally acceptable approach to trade-offs in rationing scarce health care resources should satisfy the following conditions (Purtillo, 1999):

- There should be a demonstrable need that the trade-off is necessary; the burden of proof is on those who propose the trade-off.
- There should be no choice other than the trade-off.
- All affected individuals should participate in the decision-making process, either directly or through the representatives of groups.
- Beneficial services withheld should be proportional to the actual scarcity that exists.

This approach to trade-offs is consistent with African community-oriented ethical outlooks in which the individual is understood to be embedded in a web of social relationships and interdependence (Gyekye, 1997). When considering trade-offs in the context of endemic disease and public health needs, African countries face serious dilemmas. African community-focused, "common good" standards of ethics may influence and inform trade-off decisions. As societies differ in the degree of ethical importance they place on either individual interests or the common good and the interests of communities, a range of value systems must be respected and understood.

The micro-level imperative is grounded in international standards for the practice of medicine, including the physician's duty to "act in the patient's best interest when providing medical care" (WMA, 2006, Duties of Physicians to Patients). Even at the micro level, resource allocation trade-offs sometimes occur between individual patients, in which case an additional ethical responsibility for fairness arises. According to the WMA's Declaration on the Rights of the Patient, in "circumstances where a choice must be made between potential patients for a particular treatment that is in limited supply, all such patients are entitled to a fair selection procedure for that treatment. That choice must be based on medical criteria and made without discrimination" (Williams et al., 2009, p. 70; WMA, 2005, Principle E). The moral basis for requiring fair procedure extends to the requirement for justice at the meso and macro levels, where the access of individuals, communities, and populations to potentially life-saving HIV/AIDS services is subject to the decisions of public officials and other institutional actors.

At any of the three levels of decision making, when people whose needs exceed available resources have approximately the same clinical status or risk exposure, medical criteria alone are insufficient to guide resource allocation decisions, as will often be the case with needs for HIV/AIDS prevention, treatment, and care. In these situations, compliance with the WMA's directive that choices must be based on medical criteria and made without discrimination (Williams, 2009; WMA, 2005) is necessary but not sufficient to reach an ethically sound decision. Donors, national laws, ministries of health, local health departments, managers, hospital ethics committees where they exist, and health care professionals all make resource allocation decisions using a variety of additional criteria. The criteria in use may be explicit, as are those of some governments, or may be implicit in the choices practitioners make. Decisions governed by implicit criteria can be arbitrary, often leading to inequity and inefficiency (Rosen et al., 2005). This is one of the reasons why, from a moral point of view, the process of decision making for resource allocation must incorporate robust safeguards not only against discrimination, but also against arbitrary or self-serving exercises of power (see Figure 6-1 for Joint United Nations Programme on HIV/AIDS [UNAIDS] guidance on ethical and equitable provision of treatment). This issue is addressed further below in the discussion of procedural justice.

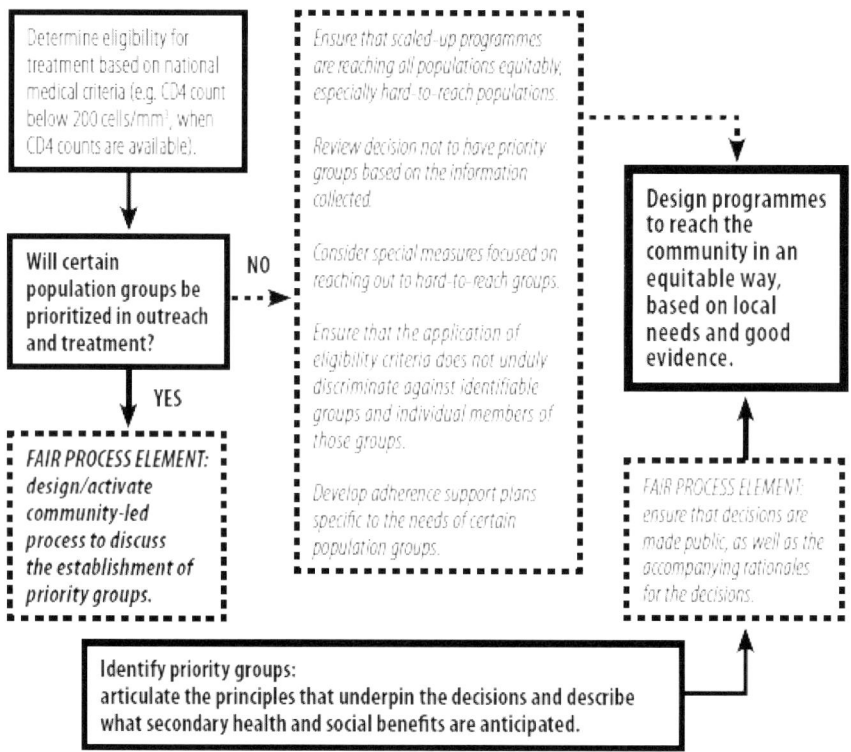

FIGURE 6-1 Roadmap for ethical and equitable provision of treatment.
NOTE: The World Health Organization's (WHO's) updated 2010 guidelines recommend eligibility for treatment at a CD4 count of 350 cells/μL.
SOURCE: UNAIDS/WHO, 2004.

Equal Moral Status

Respect for individuals' equal moral status requires fair decision making even in the face of scarcity. Each patient has an equal claim to fair decision-making procedures on the part of physicians, and each member of society has an equal claim to just treatment by institutions and the state. Equal moral status is recognized in the Universal Declaration of Human Rights (UDHR): "All human beings are born free and equal in dignity and rights" (UN, 1948).

Policy makers do not necessarily violate the principle of equal moral status by selecting certain groups—such as health workers or mothers of young children—for priority on the grounds of their expected contributions to society. However, priorities must be established through a fair process that (1) includes all stakeholders; (2) is publicly transparent, enforceable, and revisable; and (3) is founded defining efficient intervention packages for the most at-risk groups (UNAIDS, 2009).

African governments should be encouraged to adopt and apply the internationally established principles for ethical decision making in the HIV/AIDS context described above. The challenge ahead is how African health professionals, institutional leaders, and civil society can take responsibility for ethical decision making in the face of poor governance, corruption, military rule, armed conflict, civil unrest, dictatorship, and other adversities. The following section explores strategies for ensuring ethical decision-making capacity for HIV/AIDS policy and programming in Africa.

BUILDING ETHICAL DECISION-MAKING CAPACITY FOR HIV/AIDS POLICY AND PROGRAMMING IN AFRICA

Experience with and understanding of local conditions are essential components of ethical decision-making capacity. Ministries of health, national AIDS councils, and other authorities in African countries hard hit by HIV/AIDS have already had to make decisions under severely challenging circumstances for years. What lessons have they learned from this experience, and what can be done to document and disseminate these lessons? The following discussion should be considered alongside the existing base of decision-making experience in Africa. Key areas of inquiry include procedural justice in specific African contexts; which responsible parties are involved in decision-making processes and what capacities they require for ethically informed decisions; capacity building to support ethical decision making; programs in ethics and human rights currently offered in Africa; an "all-of-government" approach to health in the form of interministerial committees; and the inclusion of socially disadvantaged groups in HIV/AIDS prevention, treatment, and care efforts.

Procedural Justice in Specific African Contexts

The principle of the equal moral status of individuals requires that policy makers avoid arbitrary or capricious distinctions that discriminate against individuals and groups. Trade-offs in resource allocation can be understood as problems of *distributive justice*, defined as "fair, equitable, and appropriate distribution determined by justified norms that structure the terms of social cooperation" (Beauchamp and Childress, 2009, p. 226). Distributive justice has two complementary aspects: *substantive* justice and *procedural* justice.

Substantive justice deals with the content of allocation decisions, ensuring fair distribution of scarce resources. It requires fairness in allocating benefits and burdens in society. *Procedural* justice deals with fairness in the process of decision making. A focus on procedural justice is helpful especially when there is no reasonable prospect of consensus on substantive principles to guide resource allocation, as is likely to be the case in the trade-offs involved in HIV/AIDS-related decision making in resource-constrained African countries.

Norman Daniels' Accountability for Reasonableness (A4R) framework identifies four necessary conditions for procedural justice (Daniels, 2008):

- Publicity condition—decisions and rationales are publicly accessible.
- Relevance condition—rationales appeal to evidence, reasons, and principles accepted as relevant by fair-minded stakeholders.
- Revision and appeals condition—mechanisms and opportunities exist to challenge decisions, resolve disputes, and revise and improve policies in light of new evidence or arguments.
- Regulative condition—decision-making processes are regulated, either voluntarily or publicly, to enforce the above three conditions.

For example, A4R in "patient and site selection in the global effort to scale up ARTs for HIV/AIDS in low-income, high-prevalence countries" focuses on four issues: cost recovery for ART, medical eligibility criteria, siting of treatment facilities, and priority to special groups (Daniels, 2008, pp. 274–292). More broadly, Daniels and colleagues have developed an evidence-based policy tool called Benchmarks of Fairness for analyzing the effects of health policies on equity, efficiency, and accountability in developing countries, which has been tested in Cameroon, Ecuador, Guatemala, Thailand, and Zambia (Daniels, 2006; Daniels et al., 2000, 2005).

Youngkong and colleagues reviewed 18 empirical studies of priority setting for health interventions in developing countries, including South Africa, Tanzania, Burkina Faso, Ghana, and Uganda (Youngkong et al., 2009). Several of these studies employed the A4R model, but other models were also used:

- Lasry and colleagues (2008) describe a "decision support system" specifically aimed at local government agencies, nongovernmental organizations (NGOs), or public health institutions currently offering HIV/AIDS programs in a low-income community and illustrate its use in the context of the KwaDukuza Primary Health Care Clinic near Durban, South Africa. Kapiriri and Martin (2010) propose a framework, derived partly from qualitative research, to support practical planning and evaluation of priority-setting efforts in low- and middle-income countries.
- Kapiriri and Martin (2007) argue that to improve priority setting, it is necessary to describe current practices (while remaining aware that they are "value laden and political") and to identify the institutions and groups that have legitimacy (i.e., moral authority) so they can be empowered through training, access to tools and evidence, and legal mandates.

The achievement of procedural justice in practice depends not only on the use of a fair decision-making process but also on the secure existence of supportive political and legal institutions. These institutions are characterized below in terms of three "mandates" of procedural justice.

Mandate 1: An Informed Civil Society

According to UNAIDS, civil society speaks with many voices and represents many different perspectives (UNAIDS, 2010). Civil society is broadly defined to include HIV/AIDS service organizations; groups of people living with HIV/AIDS; youth organizations; women's organizations; businesses; trade unions; professional and scientific organizations; sports organizations; international development NGOs; and a broad spectrum of religions and faith-based organizations, both global and at the country level.

Given the diversity of civil society organizations (CSOs) within the health sector, it is not surprising that, at times, these CSOs represent competing interests as well as competitors for funding, human resources, and other important assets. While competition is of obvious value in promoting institutional performance, it also tends to discourage collaboration and risks undue duplication or dispersion of efforts (Advisory Group on Civil Society and Aid Effectiveness, 2007). Despite these potential drawbacks, CSOs can and have mobilized, empowered, and supported community responses to the HIV/AIDS epidemic. For this reason, UNAIDS and others have identified civil society as playing key roles in the response to the HIV/AIDS epidemic in countries around the world.

For CSOs to be successful, they must be fully engaged in decision-making processes. They must have access to full information and to decision-making processes, as well as the right to challenge the decisions that are made. An example is the Treatment Action Campaign, formed in 1998 in South Africa. Its purpose is to challenge unjust decisions concerning the allocation of health resources through the civil society sector. Most well known is a successful constitutional challenge before the South African Constitutional Court, which required the government to grant greater access to treatment for the prevention of mother-to-child HIV transmission (Heywood, 2003).

If procedural justice in developing countries depends upon the accountability of civil society, what then does civil society depend upon? Civil society cannot sustain itself without serious long-term funding strategies, such as those called for in the recommendations at the end of this chapter. The desired capabilities of African CSOs are not expected to be in place today, but to be built over the next decade. When the need arises to ration or fairly distribute a scarce medical resource such as ART, the lack of procedural justice can lead to chaos. Therefore, a systematic process for procedural justice is needed. Long-term procedural justice and accountability in African countries with high HIV/AIDS burdens and few resources, as in all countries, will depend upon civil society and its ability to hold governments accountable.

Mandate 2: Legal Capacity and Capability

The second mandate of procedural justice is legal capacity and capability. If decisions made are unethical and unfair, civil society must be able to challenge them. To this end, countries must follow the rule of law; operate honestly and transparently; and welcome the input of a diverse, well-informed community. Without the rule of law, particularly law incorporating the framework of human rights, it is difficult to achieve procedural justice (Heywood, 2010).

In another illustration from South Africa, civil society fought long for a new constitution that included social and economic rights. The South African constitution states that everyone has a right to access to health care services, and that the state must take reasonable legislative and other measures to progressively realize the right to access to health care services (Heywood, 2010).

Mandate 3: Shared Governance

Globally, institutions of shared governance are organizations that sit together and take responsibility for decision making around resource allocation. Although these institutions do exist, this does not mean that government abdicates responsibility. In the case of global funding for HIV/AIDS programs, NGOs and CSOs, international organizations, and national governments should all be involved in the decision-making process (Heywood, 2010).

National AIDS councils, prevalent in many African countries, illustrate shared governance. These councils often encompass a range of stakeholders including public officials, professional organizations, and NGOs. They have a variety of powers, either binding or advisory (Heywood, 2010).

Responsible Parties and Required Capacities

Taking a long-term perspective on the pursuit of procedural justice is warranted in light of the complex political and institutional components of real-world priority setting. Who *is* exerting influence, who *ought* to be exerting influence, and what practical steps can be taken to bring the two more into line? Time will be required to build an accurate understanding of the influences at work in particular decision-making contexts across many different countries and localities where resource streams are of varying origins, levels, and degrees of predictability, and where the HIV/AIDS epidemic takes different forms and has different impacts.

Meanwhile, it is possible to identify and empower stakeholders in particular settings who should have more influence than they actually do. For example, when a sample of health workers in Uganda was asked to rank actors by actual versus ideal influence on priority setting, respondents identified patients and the general public as those who should have more influence than they actually do, as compared with donors and politicians, whom respondents viewed as having excessive influence (Kapiriri et al., 2004). A parallel, alternative approach is to identify relatively enduring processes through which resource allocation decisions are actually made and to enhance the ethical capacity (relative to HIV/AIDS policy and programming) of already-empowered actors. The range of such actors might include local health service providers, local health system managers, HIV/AIDS program implementers, civil society (community-based organizations and NGOs), traditional leaders, local public officials, academic institutions, national public officials, regional organizations, and the media (to promote responsible and balanced reporting of information in support of participatory democracy).

Some countries have already developed approaches to ethical decision making in the face of scarce resources, both fiscal and human. In Cameroon, for example, a physician's choice of a treatment protocol must be submitted to a therapeutics committee for discussion and approval. A weekly or bimonthly meeting is held with all relevant personnel, including physicians, paramedics, social workers, and possibly community relay agents, to discuss, revise, or approve the protocol. The members of the therapeutics committee receive training prior to their service (Eboko et al., 2010). At the community level, governments should consider creating multidisciplinary treatment and care committees, similar to those in Cameroon, to guide practitioner-driven decisions. These committees would carefully review, modify, and approve treatment and care protocols for persons with HIV/AIDS.

Capacity Building to Support Ethical Decision Making

Several key questions arise regarding capacity building for institutions, groups, and individuals to support effective leadership and participation in the sorts of decision-making processes that would help realize conditions of procedural justice. First, to what extent, and for whom, is formal training in ethics required? Training would be valuable both to meet immediate needs and to contribute to long-term capacity building. What are the options for providing such training? How should curricula be designed? How can culturally and historically relevant content be developed? Possibilities include ethics courses or modules in degree programs for nursing, medicine, public health, government, management, and media, as well as ethics components in continuing education programs for active professionals. To address these issues, partnerships among academic institutions, government, and professional organizations should be explored. Second, it is possible to identify a set of core competencies integrating all the factors relevant to sound decision making—not only ethics but also budgeting and management, evidence assessment, health policy analysis, and communications. Assuming it would be rare and costly for any one person to master all of the requisite competencies, what can organizations do to distribute areas of competency across personnel teams? Third, what inputs are needed to support sound decision making—such as interpretations of scientific evidence, or data for program monitoring and evaluation—and how can they be supplied in a regular and timely manner? Fourth, how can ethical and evidential considerations be effectively communicated, as needed, among local, district, national, and regional decision makers? Fifth, to the extent that resources come from foreign donors, how can institutions be constructed to gain donors' trust so that donors will be willing to relinquish some control over resource allocation decisions?

Programs in Ethics and Human Rights Currently Offered in Africa

An extensive literature search reveals that while several programs within and outside of educational institutions include ethics and/or human rights, they are directed mainly at ethics of health-related research. Funders of ethics activities in Africa include the United Nations Educational, Scientific and Cultural Organization (UNESCO), the Wellcome Trust, the Fogarty Center, and the European Union. UNESCO has developed an extensive database of ethics teaching programs on the continent. At the postgraduate level, only three African institutions have developed capacity-building programs in ethics and human rights that do not focus mainly on research.[3] At the undergraduate level, the Health Professions Council of South Africa (HPCSA) has developed a core curriculum in bioethics, human rights, and health law that is integrated into health sciences curricula. The following core competencies are required by HPCSA to qualify health care practitioners:

- Show respect for patients and colleagues without prejudice, with an understanding and an appreciation of their diversities of background and opportunity, language, and culture.
- Strive to improve patient care, reduce inequalities in health care delivery, and optimize the use of health care resources in our society.
- Use his or her professional capabilities to contribute to the community as well as to individual patient welfare.
- Demonstrate awareness, through action or in writing, of the legal and ethical responsibilities involved in individual patient care and the provision of care to populations.
- Consider the impact of health care on the environment and the impact of the environment on health (The Committee on Human Rights Ethics and Professional Practice, 2006, p. 5).

---

[3] Two of these programs are in South Africa and one in the Malawi College of Medicine. The University of Cape Town offers an extensive Train the Trainers Program on Health and Human Rights, and the University of Witwatersrand runs a Masters in Bioethics and Health Law program whose Research Ethics module, while compulsory, represents just 10 percent of the program.

It is important that students be exposed to critical thinking and ethical analysis and reasoning and provided with pertinent resources to develop these skills as early in their training as possible. These skills can then be used to develop professionalism that will help students be prepared when they eventually face complex decisions in a range of situations, from the patient's bedside to policy-level decision making in the health ministry.

Finally, while it is important to develop programs that extend beyond research ethics, it is necessary to bear in mind that the HIV/AIDS epidemic has rendered Africa fertile ground for the global proliferation of clinical research, including multicenter, international, and pharmaceutical studies. Research must continue to serve the health needs of the continent. It must always be ethical, protecting the rights and well-being of participants. Research participants are often vulnerable, burdened by multiple health conditions, poverty, illiteracy, and lack of full access to health care. These conditions, together with the several examples of exploitation to which the continent has been subjected, underscore the importance of maintaining high ethical standards. Currently, the research ethics committee (REC) process serves this protective function. If this function is to be carried out with commitment, however, it will incur financial costs, and funders, including PEPFAR and the Global Fund, must consider developing ethics capacities in this arena.

While most countries in Africa use international benchmarks for their research participant programs, capacity to implement these benchmarks varies among RECs within and among countries. Programs should be developed to address these shortfalls, together with monitoring and evaluation. National and regional RECs, for example, could be constituted to address these concerns.

Interministerial Committees

A comprehensive approach to the management of HIV/AIDS will include ensuring the basic survival needs of the people in a country, thereby addressing the delivery of some of the social determinants of health (Gostin, 2007, 2008). Health cannot be achieved if it is viewed as a silo, with the only responsible and accountable people being ministers of health and their designees. Some of the fundamental requisites for meeting basic survival needs are well-functioning health systems, essential medicines and vaccines, clean air, clean water, diet and nutrition, sanitation, sewage, and pest control, which can go a long way toward alleviating poverty. However, social, economic, cultural, and behavioral determinants (e.g., living and working conditions, mental health, spiritual well-being, physical environment, personal health practices, capacity, culture, and discriminatory practices) impact health (WHO, 1986). Also required, therefore, is a broader view of health needs based on social determinants that incorporates psychosocial and justice issues. Access to health facilities is necessary as well, in turn requiring attention to adequate transport. Finally, health is influenced substantially by choices people make about how to live their lives. For these choices to be well informed, people must have access to education and information.

Accordingly, in the committee's judgment, building ethical decision-making capacity requires multisectoral and multidisciplinary collaboration. National governments should consider incorporating professionals with training in ethics into interministerial committees that address all issues affecting the public's health, analogous to the South African Ministerial Council on Innovation now being considered.

Inclusion of Socially Disadvantaged Groups in HIV/ AIDS Prevention, Treatment, and Care Efforts

Criminalization of same-sex behavior in certain African countries and its adverse impacts on efforts to address the HIV/AIDS epidemic are of serious concern. The committee welcomes efforts to counteract the criminalization movement, such as the new United Nations Development Programme (UNDP)/ UNAIDS Global Commission on HIV and the Law.

The committee raises this issue both as a component of procedural justice and as a concern in its own right. In some countries, the epidemic is concentrated among groups whose behavior is criminalized or stigmatized, such as men who have sex with men, commercial sex workers, and injecting drug users. Members of these groups are at heightened risk of exposure to HIV infection. Moreover, preventive interventions could be delivered to them very cost-effectively (Hecht et al., 2009). Yet political will to reach out to these individuals with preventive services is often lacking among both governments and donors, and some governments are actively hostile to these groups. What are some viable options for representing their interests fairly in decision making about HIV/AIDS policy and programming? Similar questions apply to girls and women who lack the means to negotiate safe sex. In general, the political constituency for preventive services is meager. How can the political will to pursue prevention efforts be strengthened in accordance with the evidentially demonstrable need for them? How can the broader public health impact of adequate preventive measures be appreciated, perhaps from the viewpoint of enlightened self-interest among members of society at large, without scapegoating groups already suffering from a concentrated epidemic?

While socially disadvantaged groups are particularly vulnerable, so, too, are children, particularly girls, who have lost one or both parents and have little support, most of whom have to stop going to school (Case et al., 2004). They are placed on a usually irreversible downward trajectory that can include transactional sex and a high risk of HIV/AIDS. Much has been written about AIDS orphans, and PEPFAR focuses on this group. However, the needs of children made vulnerable by HIV/AIDS will continue to grow, requiring special attention in ethical decision making relating to their health, education, and well-being. Prevention efforts targeting children have the potential for long-term positive effects. Ethical guidance is needed to ensure that all vulnerable children are reached, not just those already affected by HIV/AIDS.[4]

The ethical imperative of equal moral status of individuals and the mandates of procedural justice are largely being ignored with regard to socially disadvantaged groups and vulnerable children. Major opportunities for prevention are also missed, as these groups are less likely than others to access HIV/AIDS services. The UNAIDS International Guidelines on HIV/AIDS and Human Rights (see Annex 6-1) delineate the necessary capacities for states to protect these groups and offer a legal framework for their protection, including antidiscrimination laws. However, many countries do not comply with these guidelines.

RECOMMENDATIONS

The committee concludes that many key decision makers in Africa need assistance in developing the capacity for ethical decision making with respect to policies, programs, and resource allocation for HIV/AIDS in their populations. Core competencies for ethical decision making need to be defined in such areas as budgeting, management, evidence assessment, communications, and health policy analysis. Insufficient capacity exists to deal with counterethical pressures from powerful actors. In many cases, government officials also need assistance in developing accountability and competence for their decisions, particularly with reference to priority setting and fair allocation of scarce resources. Therefore, the committee offers the following recommendations.

Recommendation 6-1: *Enable and reinforce capacity for ethical decision making.* Donors and governments should help build capacity for ethical decision making by adequately funding education and training in the disciplines of ethics, human rights, and pertinent aspects of the law. This training should include both educational and implementation components.

Recommendation 6-2: *Donors and governments should support civil society organizations where they exist and help develop them in other places over time.* As a first step, the focus should be on procedural justice. Therefore, U.S. government agencies, including the State Department, USAID, and the Department of Health and Human Services, should provide technical and financial support to recipients of their health assistance for the establishment of effective mechanisms for procedural justice, including transparency, accountability, and responsibility.

---

[4] A discussion of this especially vulnerable population and some efforts to ameliorate their lot can be found in the Institute of Medicine reports (IOM, 2007, 2010).

Recommendation 6-3: *Professionals with training in ethics should be incorporated into multisectoral teams.* To increase the capacity for ethical decision making at the national level, professionals with training in ethics should be incorporated into national government multisectoral teams that include ministries of health, finance, and education, as well as other government ministries whose work is relevant to HIV/AIDS; civil society organizations; educational institutions; professional organizations; and nongovernmental organizations.

REFERENCES

Advisory Group on Civil Society and Aid Effectiveness. 2007. Civil society and aid effectiveness: Issues paper. http://www.oecd.org/dataoecd/59/11/39499142.pdf (accessed November 1, 2010).

African Union. 2003. *Maputo declaration on HIV/AIDS, tuberculosis, malaria, and other related infectious diseases.* http://www.africa-union.org/ root/ AU/ Conferences/ Past/2006/March/ SA/ Mar6/ Maputo_Declaration_HIV-AIDSTB.pdf (accessed August 10, 2010).

Beauchamp, T. L., and J. S. Childress. 2009. *Principles of biomedical ethics,* 6th ed. New York: Oxford University Press.

Case, A., C. Paxson, and J. Ableidinger. 2004. Orphans in Africa: Parental death, poverty, and school enrollment. *Demography* 41(3):483-508.

The Committee on Human Rights Ethics and Professional Practice. 2006. *Core curriculum on human rights, ethics and medical law for health care practitioners.* Pretoria: Health Professions Council of South Africa.

Daniels, N. 2004. *How to achieve fair distribution of ARTs in 3 by 5: Fair process and legitimacy in patient selection.* Geneva: WHO.

———. 2006. Toward ethical review of health system transformations. *American Journal of Public Health* 96(3):447-451.

———. 2008. *Just health: Meeting health needs fairly.* New York: Cambridge University Press.

Daniels, N., J. Bryant, R. A. Castano, O. G. Dantes, K. S. Khan, and S. Pannarunothai. 2000. Benchmarks of fairness for health care reform: A policy tool for developing countries. *Bulletin of the World Health Organization* 78(6):740-750.

Daniels, N., W. Flores, S. Pannarunothai, P. N. Ndumbe, J. H. Bryant, T. J. Ngulube, and Y. K. Wang. 2005. An evidence-based approach to benchmarking the fairness of health-sector reform in developing countries. *Bulletin of the World Health Organization* 83(7):534-540.

Eboko, F., C. Abé, and C. Laurent. 2010. *Accès décentralisé au traitement du VIH/sida: Évaluation de l'expérience camerounaise.* Agence Nationale de recerches: sur le sida et les hipatites virales. Paris: ANRS.

Gostin, L. O. 2007. Meeting the survival needs of the world's least healthy people: A proposed model for global health governance. *Journal of the American Medical Association* 298(2):225-228.

———. 2008. Meeting basic survival needs of the world's least healthy people: Toward a framework convention on global health. *Georgetown Law Journal* 96(2):331-392.

———. 2009. *Public health law: Power, duty, restraint,* 2nd ed. Berkeley: University of California Press.

Gyekye, K. 1997. *Tradition and modernity: Philosophical reflections on the African experience.* New York: Oxford University Press.

Haacker, M. 2009. Financing HIV/AIDS programs in sub-Saharan Africa. *Health Affairs* 28(6): 1606-1616.

Hecht, R., L. Bollinger, J. Stover, W. McGreevey, F. Muhib, C. E. Madavo, and D. de Ferranti. 2009. Critical choices in financing the response to the global HIV/AIDS pandemic. *Health Affairs* 28(6):1591-1605.

Heywood, M. 2003. Preventing mother-to-child HIV transmission in South Africa: Background, strategies and outcomes of the Treatment Action Campaign's case against the Minister of Health. *South African Journal on Human Rights* 19(2):38.

———. 2010. Presentation to the IOM committee on envisioning a strategy to prepare for the long-term burden of HIV/AIDS: African needs and U.S. interests. Pretoria, South Africa, April 12, 2010.

IOM (Institute of Medicine). 2005. *Scaling up treatment for the global AIDS pandemic: Challenges and opportunities.* Washington, DC: The National Academies Press.

———. 2007. *PEPFAR implementation: Progress and promise.* Washington, DC: The National Academies Press.

———. 2010. *Strategic approach to the evaluation of programs implemented under the Tom Lantos and Henry J. Hyde U.S. Global Leadership against HIV/AIDS, Tuberculosis, and Malaria Reauthorization Act of 2008.* Washington, DC: The National Academies Press.

Kapiriri, L., T. Arnesen, and O. F. Norheim. 2004. Is cost-effectiveness analysis preferred to severity of disease as the main guiding principle in priority setting in resource poor settings? The case of Uganda. *Cost Effectiveness and Resource Allocation* 2.

Kapiriri, L., and D. K. Martin. 2007. A strategy to improve priority setting in developing countries. *Health Care Analysis* 15(3):159-167.

———. 2010. Successful priority setting in low and middle income countries: A framework for evaluation. *Health Care Analysis* 18:129-147.

Lasry, A., M. Carter, and G. Zaric. 2008. S4HARA: System for HIV/AIDS resource allocation. *Cost Effectiveness and Resource Allocation* 6(1):7.

Macklin, R. 2004. *Ethics and equity in access to HIV treatment: 3 by 5 initiative.* Geneva: WHO.

Mandaville, A. 2007. *MCC and the long term goal of deepening democracy.* Washington, DC: Millennium Challenge Corporation.

Organisation of African Unity (OAU). 2000. Lome declaration: Declarations of the decisions adopted by the thirty-sixth ordinary session of the assembly of heads of state and government. In *AHG/ Decl. 1 (XXXVI).* Lome, Togo.

———. 2001. *Abuja declaration on HIV/AIDS, tuberculosis, and other related diseases.* Abuja, Nigeria.

Project HOPE. 2009. The difficult but necessary choices in fighting HIV/AIDS. *Health Affairs* 28(6):1575-1577.

Purtillo, R. 1999. Distributive justice: Clinical sources of claims for health care. In *Ethical dimensions for the health professions,* 3rd ed. Philadelphia: Saunders Company. Pp. 251-266.

Rosen, S., I. Sanne, A. Collier, and J. L. Simon. 2005. Hard choices: Rationing antiretroviral therapy for HIV/AIDS in Africa. *The Lancet* 365(9456):354-356.

UN (United Nations). 1948. *Universal declaration of human rights.* Paper read at general assembly of the United Nations. http://www.eduhi.at/dl/Universal_Declaration_of_Human_Rights.pdf (accessed November 1, 2010).

———. 1966. *International covenant on economic, social and cultural rights.* Paper read at general assembly of the United Nations. http://www2.ohchr.org/english/law/cescr.htm (accessed August 2, 2010).

———. 2001. Declaration of commitment on HIV/AIDS. In *S-26/2.* General Assembly. http://www. un.org/ga/aids/docs/aress262.pdf (accessed August 2, 2010).

———. 2003. *Convention on the Rights of the Child.* New York: UN.

———. 2005. World summit outcome. In *60/1.* General Assembly. http://unpan1.un.org/intradoc/ groups/public/documents/un/unpan021752.pdf (accessed August 2, 2010).

UN Economic and Social Council. 2000. *The right to the highest attainable standard of health.* Geneva: UN.

———. 2004. *Economic, social and cultural rights: The right of everyone to the enjoyment of the highest attainable standard of physical and mental health. Report of the Special Rapporteur, Paul Hunt.* Geneva: UN.

———. 2005. *Economic, social and cultural rights: Report of the Special Rapporteur on the right of everyone to the enjoyment of the highest attainable standard of physical and mental health, Paul Hunt.* Geneva: UN.

UNAIDS (The Joint United Nations Programme on HIV/AIDS). 2009. *Update on the impact of the economic crisis: HIV prevention and treatment programmes.* http://data.unaids.org/pub/Report/2010/economiccrisisandhivandaids61_en.pdf (accessed August 12, 2010).

———. 2010. *Civil society.* http://www.unaids.org/en/Partnerships/Civil+society/default.asp (accessed November 1, 2010).

UNAIDS/WHO. 2004. *Guidance on ethics and equitable access to HIV treatment and care.* Geneva: WHO.

WHO (World Health Organization). 1986. Ottawa charter for health promotion. In *WHO/HPR/HEP/95.1.* Ottawa, Canada: First International Conference on Health Promotion.

Williams, J. R. 2009. *World Medical Association Medical Ethics Manual,* 2nd ed. Ferney-Voltaire Cedex: WMA.

Williams, T. P., M. Vibbert, L. Mitchell, and R. Serwanga. 2009. Health and human rights of children affected by HIV/AIDS in urban Boston and rural Uganda: A cross-cultural partnership. *International Social Work* 52(4):539-545.

WMA (World Medical Association). 2005. *Declaration on the rights of the patient.* http://www.wma.net/en/30publications/10policies/l4/index.html (accessed June 1, 2010).

———. 2006. *International code of medical ethics.* http://www.wma.net/en/30publications/10policies/c8/index.html (accessed June 1, 2010).

Youngkong, S., L. Kapiriri, and R. Baltussen. 2009. Setting priorities for health interventions in developing countries: A review of empirical studies. *Tropical Medicine and International Health* 14(8):930-939.

ANNEX 6-1
INTERNATIONAL GUIDELINES ON
HIV/AIDS AND HUMAN RIGHTS

The UNAIDS 2006 International Guidelines on HIV/AIDS and Human Rights (consolidating Consultations from September 1996 and July 2002) are as follows:

1. States should establish an effective national framework for their response to HIV/AIDS which ensures a coordinated, participatory, transparent and accountable approach, integrating HIV/AIDS policy and program responsibilities across all branches of government.
2. States should ensure, through political and financial support, that community consultation occurs in all phases of HIV/AIDS policy design, program implementation and evaluation and that community organizations are enabled to carry out their activities, including in the field of ethics, law and human rights, effectively.
3. States should review and reform public health laws to ensure that they adequately address public health issues raised by HIV/AIDS, that their provisions applicable to casually transmitted diseases are not inappropriately applied to HIV/AIDS and that they are consistent with international human rights obligations.
4. States should review and reform criminal laws and correctional systems to ensure that they are consistent with international human rights obligations and are not misused in the context of HIV/AIDS or targeted against vulnerable groups.
5. States should enact or strengthen anti-discrimination and other protective laws that protect vulnerable groups, people living with HIV/AIDS and people with disabilities from discrimination in both the public and private sectors, ensure privacy and confidentiality and ethics in research involving human subjects, emphasize education and conciliation, and provide for speedy and effective administrative and civil remedies.
6. States should enact legislation to provide for the regulation of HIV-related goods, services and information, so as to ensure widespread availability of qualitative prevention measures and services, adequate HIV prevention and care information and safe and effective medication at an affordable price.
7. States should implement and support legal support services that will educate people affected by HIV/AIDS about their rights, provide free legal services to enforce those rights, develop expertise on HIV-related legal issues and utilize means of protection in addition to the courts, such as offices of ministries of justice, ombudsmen, health complaint units and human rights commissions.

8. States, in collaboration with and through the community, should promote a supportive and enabling environment for women, children and other vulnerable groups by addressing underlying prejudices and inequalities through community dialogue, specially designed social and health services and support to community groups.

9. States should promote the wide and ongoing distribution of creative education, training and media programs explicitly designed to change attitudes of discrimination and stigmatization associated with HIV/AIDS to understanding and acceptance.

10. States should ensure that government and private sectors develop codes of conduct regarding HIV/AIDS issues that translate human rights principles into codes of professional responsibility and practice, with accompanying mechanisms to implement and enforce those codes.

11. States should ensure monitoring and enforcement mechanisms to guarantee the protection of HIV-related human rights, including those of people living with HIV/AIDS, their families and communities.

12. States should cooperate through all relevant programs and agencies of the United Nations system, including the Joint United Nations Programme on HIV/AIDS, to share knowledge and experience concerning HIV-related human rights issues and should ensure effective mechanisms to protect human rights in the context of HIV/AIDS at the international level.

Appendix A

Projecting the Burden of HIV/AIDS

In planning for a long-term response to the HIV/AIDS epidemic in Africa in the coming decade, the global community needs to ask how reliable projections for different variables can be. How well can we project the future course of the epidemic? How well can we predict the impact of treatment interventions? How well can we predict the impact of prevention efforts? How well can we predict the epidemic's social, demographic, and financial burdens? How well can we predict the financial resources available to combat HIV/AIDS?

EPIDEMIOLOGICAL PROJECTIONS

The ability to predict the course and impact of the HIV/AIDS epidemic is reasonably good over the short term because the current situation evolves gradually, driven by biological or other relatively well-understood processes (e.g., those already infected progress to AIDS). Over the longer term, less predictable factors could alter the risk of HIV infection and the resources available to combat the epidemic. Eventually, game-changing technologies, such as a cure or vaccine, may exist, but the availability of resources will continue to impact populations' access to them. One of the greatest uncertainties is the availability of treatment for those who need it, which will determine the numbers of deaths and impact the incidence of new infections.

In the absence of antiretroviral therapy (ART), the progression of HIV from infection to AIDS and death is a slow process with a median time to death of 11 years, with survival depending on age and other factors (Todd et al., 2007). Most of those progressing to AIDS and needing treatment over the next decade are already infected with the virus. Unlike many other aspects of this epidemic, the need for treatment is predictable. The number of people on treatment over time is a function of the rates of diagnosis, treatment initiation, and survival on treatment. These rates are also predictable given assumptions about investment in treatment programs and the organization of those programs. The scale and success of treatment will determine the impact of treatment interventions. The social and economic burden of HIV/AIDS will depend upon the success of treatment programs, as well as the efforts undertaken to care for those affected. In contrast, the accumulation of new infections over time is more difficult to predict since it will depend on changing patterns of risk in the population, which in turn are influenced by demographic, cultural, and social phenomena, as well as the impact of preventive interventions.

Over the course of the epidemic, some patterns of risk behavior will likely change, making it difficult to link the current observed prevalence of HIV to measures of risk behavior with precision. Furthermore, the sensitive, private, and often stigmatized behaviors that place many at risk of acquiring HIV may not be accurately reported in surveys (Fenton et al., 2001; Slaymaker, 2004), making it difficult to relate incidence to behavior and predict how changes in behavior will influence incidence (Garnett et al., 2006). A straightforward assumption is that trends in HIV incidence will continue in the future. With incidence trends stable, future prevalence will be determined largely by the future expansion of ART, which has both direct and indirect effects on prevalence. The direct effect of ART expansion is to lengthen the lives of people with HIV, which consequently increases prevalence. ART also has several possible indirect effects on HIV prevalence, both beneficial and adverse, through its effects on transmission and therefore on incidence (see Table A-1).

In the *aids2031*[1] predictions, it is assumed that those on treatment have a reduced infectiousness (to 20 percent of the original transmission risk from an infected person to susceptible contacts) (aids2031 Consortium, 2011; Hecht et al., 2010). In formulating its baseline projections, the committee developed a model incorporating two of the biological effects from Table A-1—the reduction in transmission among those on effective ART and the increased exposure to risk caused by a longer HIV-infected lifespan. Since the degree to which the two behavioral effects in Table A-1 will manifest as treatment access increases is still unknown and will likely be responsive to national HIV/AIDS policies, the baseline model ignores these and the other indirect effects of ART on HIV transmission.[2]

Others have made projections of the impact of particular interventions over

---

[1] *aids2031* is a consortium of partners who came together to look at what has been learned about the HIV/AIDS response and consider the implications of the changing world around the HIV/AIDS pandemic *(aids2031* Consortium, 2010).

[2] The committee's model is Version 4.05 of the open-source AIDSCost projection model, available for download on the Center for Global Development website (Over, 2009).

Impacts on Infants and Children

The WHO 2010 updated pediatric ART guidelines advise that all HIV-positive children less than 24 months of age be started on ART (WHO, 2010). The number of children infected with HIV is a function of the HIV prevalence in women of reproductive age; the fertility rate of those women; whether and for how long they breastfeed infants; whether PMTCT is used; and if it is, how efficacious the regimen is in preventing vertical transmission. The infection of children can be prevented directly by implementing PMTCT interventions or indirectly by preventing the spread of HIV through women.

Young people aged 15–24 account for an estimated 45 percent of new HIV infections worldwide. Globally, the number of children younger than 15 living with HIV increased from 1.6 million in 2001 to 2.1 million in 2008. Almost 90 percent live in sub-Saharan Africa (UNAIDS, 2008; UNAIDS and WHO, 2009).

Mother-to-child, or perinatal, transmission continues to account for a substantial, although decreasing, portion of these new HIV infections in many African countries (UNAIDS and WHO, 2009). It is estimated that 90 percent of children living with HIV acquired the virus during pregnancy, birth, or breastfeeding—all forms of HIV transmission that can be prevented (UNAIDS, 2008). In Swaziland, children were estimated to account for nearly one in five (19 percent) new HIV infections in 2008 (Mngadi et al., 2009; UNAIDS and WHO, 2009). Perinatally acquired infection accounted for 15 percent of new HIV infections in Uganda in 2008 (UNAIDS and WHO, 2009; Wabwire-Mangen et al., 2009).

HIV is the underlying reason for more than one-third of all deaths in children under the age of 5 (UNAIDS, 2008). Without ART, the progression of HIV infection in children is particularly aggressive, and many children die at a young age (UNAIDS, 2008). Among infants and children exposed to HIV, access to early testing, care, and treatment is insufficient. In 2009, in 54 reporting countries, only 15 percent of children born to HIV-positive mothers received an HIV test within the first 2 months of life (WHO, 2010). ART coverage among children less than 15 years of age in 2009 was only 28 percent (up from 22 percent in 2008); a mere 35 percent of infants in need received PMTCT prophylaxis in 2009 (up from 32 percent in 2008); and the percentage of pregnant women living with HIV receiving ART for PMTCT in 2009 was 53 percent (up from 45 percent in 2008) (WHO, 2010). Globally, however, coverage for PMTCT services did rise from 10 percent in 2004 to 45 percent in 2008; the drop in new HIV infections among children in 2008 suggests that these efforts are saving lives (UNAIDS and WHO, 2009) (see Figure A-1).

The causal links from PMTCT policy to treatment needs run in both directions. Not only does PMTCT expansion reduce the number of infants needing treatment, but the choice of an ambitious "test-and-treat" strategy for ART expansion would require initiating virtually all HIV-infected expectant mothers on lifetime ART regardless of CD4 count. This strategy would involve a significant

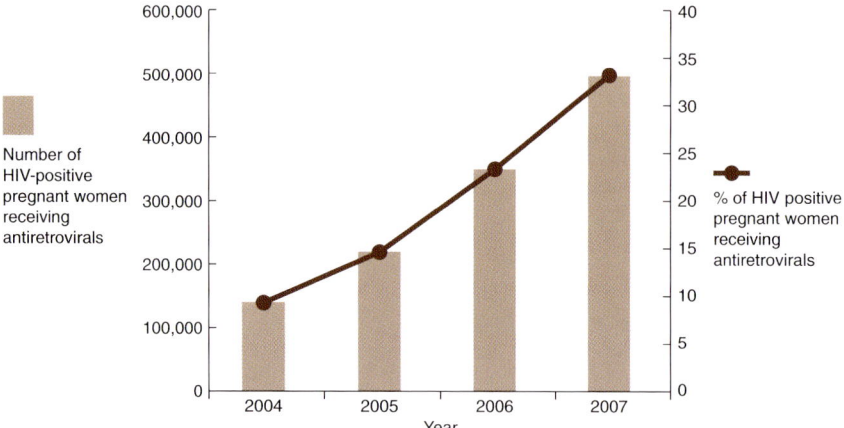

FIGURE A-1 Number and percentage of HIV-positive pregnant women receiving antiretroviral prophylaxis for PMTCT.
SOURCE: UNAIDS, 2008.

proportion of HIV-infected mothers starting therapy earlier than others and therefore remaining on treatment for a longer period of time.

AIDS orphans are defined as children who lose either a mother or father or both through HIV/AIDS-associated mortality. To predict the number of AIDS orphans, one must know the mortality rate of adults, their fertility history in the 18 years prior to death, and the survival of any children. The effort is complicated by vertical transmission of HIV leading to higher-than-background mortality in some children and the influence of HIV infection on reducing fertility. The use of ART makes it more likely that children will be born to HIV-infected mothers and less likely that they will acquire HIV infection vertically. However, ART also makes it less likely that the parent will die, and, of course, living parents decrease the societal burden of orphaned children. In general, ART should reduce the rates of orphanhood. However, a poor-quality program that delays mortality only for a short while could have the perverse effect of increasing numbers of orphans.

What Drives the Differences Among Projections?

Models include the details and assumptions required to address the questions they are designed to answer. Some models of future treatment need and patterns of survival on treatment start with an HIV-infected population and represent their declining CD4 count—either explicitly, as a function of time since infection, or using categories representing ranges of CD4 count through which individuals progress (Hallett et al., 2008; Kimmel et al., 2005; Phillips et al., 2008). Such models are useful in assessing the benefits of different treatment strategies and provide a framework for exploring the cost-effectiveness of treatments. Other models represent transmission and include the influence of treatment or behavior change on the spread of infection (Baggaley et al., 2006; Blower et al., 2005; Granich et al., 2009a). Two approaches are possible in models exploring the impact of HIV prevention interventions. The first is to use changes in proximate risk behaviors that are the intermediate endpoints measured in trials. This is a relatively conservative approach adopted in the *aids2031* models. A second approach is to assume that prevention interventions can generally have an impact reflecting an effect of "effort." (See Annex A-2 for a more thorough discussion of what drives the differences among projections.)

ECONOMIC PROJECTIONS

The committee's economic projections address the annual costs of treating a single patient, potential efficiencies, the cumulating costs of treatment, and the nature of treatment.

Annual Costs of Treating a Single Patient

The costs of treatment have been estimated in a number of different ways. One method is to seek prices for the various components of treatment (Hecht et al., 2009, 2010). Another method is to survey treatment programs and review the costs of their activities (OGAC, 2010c). A third method is to look at the overall costs and the number of people on treatment. In the estimation of treatment costs for *aids2031*, the costs include the unit costs of antiretroviral drugs, estimated as $167.65 for first-line and $1016.48 for second-line drugs based on average costs in 2007. Added to these figures are laboratory costs of $190.94 per patient per year and service delivery costs of $72.05 per patient per year for Africa; the service delivery costs are assumed to be greater in other regions. The result is an estimate of $430.64 per person per year treated (*aids2031* Costs and Financing Working Group, 2010).

The above estimate is significantly below the actual costs based on the U.S. President's Emergency Plan for AIDS Relief (PEPFAR's) survey of facilities it supports, which resulted in an estimated total mean cost of $812 per patient per year (OGAC, 2010c). Of this total, PEPFAR bore an estimated $402 per patient per year on first-line treatment, with the rest covered by other donors and national resources. The purchase of antiretroviral drugs accounted for 39 percent of costs. Of those costs captured at the facility level, 20 percent were incurred above the facility level by supervising or sponsoring organizations,[5] 36 percent were recurrent costs other than antiretroviral drugs, and only 5 percent were health system

---

[5] Comparison with Figure A-2 below suggests, and the PEPFAR facility study authors confirm, that this facility-level study captured only a small portion of costs incurred above the facility level.

investments (OGAC, 2010c). Included in these calculations are clinical staff salaries and benefits, laboratory and clinical supplies, nonantiretroviral drugs for opportunistic infections, building utilities, travel, contracted services, building renovation and construction, laboratory and clinical equipment, training, and a buffer stock of antiretroviral drugs.

These figures are somewhat puzzling when one compares the number of people treated and the overall costs reported by PEPFAR. Figure A-2 shows the average treatment costs per year per downstream PEPFAR patient computed from the Office of the Global AIDS Coordinator's (OGAC's) aggregate data (OGAC, 2010a) versus the total number of downstream patients. The best-fitting linear-in-logarithms prediction (shown as a diagonal line in the figure) suggests mild economies of scale for these national PEPFAR programs, with each 10 percent increase in scale associated with a 3 percent decline in average cost.

However, when one looks at the data, PEPFAR expenditure per patient is substantially greater than would be expected from PEPFAR's own survey of facilities, suggesting that more than half of PEPFAR's AIDS treatment expenditures are consumed before they reach the treatment site. Some of these additional costs above the facility level are justified as a contribution to the quality and efficiency of ART service delivery on the ground, while others are probably due to inadequate coordination, overly complex administrative procedures, and even fraud and abuse. The degree of efficiency in the delivery of HIV/AIDS services and the determinants of efficient, quality service delivery deserve active investiga-

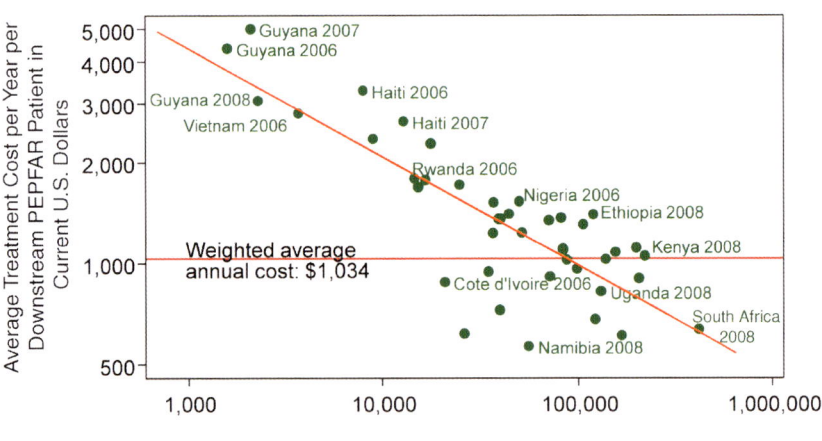

FIGURE A-2 Average unit costs of treatment reported by PEPFAR show mild economies of scale.
SOURCE: Committee analysis of OGAC data from OGAC 2010a,b.

tion. Only through an understanding of the variation in quality-adjusted efficiency across service facilities and contractors and the determinants of that variation can procurement policies be reformed to deliver more high-quality services for U.S. taxpayer dollars. PEPFAR is currently deepening its investigation of these issues, but without fully disclosing its methods or the data it is gathering at public expense. By shining a spotlight on inefficient or low-quality service providers, full public disclosure would enable improved efficiency in HIV/AIDS service delivery, thereby serving the interests of not only U.S. taxpayers but also the citizens of affected recipient countries.

The costs of treatment do not normally include the costs of counseling and testing—a necessary precursor to treatment in that it provides the diagnosis of infection and is the start of the pathway into care. However, counseling and testing could also be seen as prevention—directly if it influences the behaviors of those tested and indirectly if it improves the acceptability of the infection within the population, reducing stigma and risk. Evidence for the effect of counseling and testing on behavior is limited, with data suggesting that those diagnosed as HIV-positive reduce their risk behavior for a period of time; those diagnosed as HIV-negative do not change their behavior; and where there is couples testing, discordant couples significantly increase their condom use (Hallett et al., 2009a; Sweat et al., 2000). Further trial results powered to detect an effect of testing on HIV incidence are expected soon. Depending on these results, some portion of these testing costs should be added to the above costs of treatment, inflating the cost of treatment even more.[6]

Potential Efficiencies

Two options are available for expanding the number of people receiving ART: an increase in resources or an increase in efficiencies. The costs of antiretroviral drugs have fallen dramatically since the drugs were introduced in 1996 and currently constitute a minority of the costs of ART. To increase efficiency (i.e., decrease costs per patient), there may still be some scope for reduced drug costs, but the impact would be limited by other costs for which there may be more scope for reduction. There is a trend toward better-quality treatment with earlier initiation, viral load monitoring to ensure success, monitoring of adherence and other support services, more expensive drugs with a better profile, and second-line and salvage therapy. This trend results in increased costs per person treated, allowing fewer to receive treatment within a fixed budget. One option for achieving greater efficiencies is to make treatment simpler (UNAIDS, 2010), with

---

[6] The larger the benefits of testing for prevention, the smaller is the proportion of the costs that should be borne by treatment budgets. However, counseling and testing done to identify patients who require treatment may be less elaborate and therefore less effective at reducing risk behavior compared with counseling and testing aimed primarily at HIV prevention.

the implication in the short term (i.e., absent the development of more effective simple regimens) that the treatment would be less effective. Another option is to identify waste and inefficiencies in the organization of services.

Setting and accepting a target for the number of people receiving treatment that is in line with current treatment costs results in little incentive to reduce those costs. There is a negative correlation between the number of HIV-infected individuals in a country and the cost per person treated, suggesting modest economies of scale with respect to the magnitude of a national AIDS treatment program. However, further expansion will entail two sources of diseconomies as existing infrastructure and human resources are pushed to their limits. First, within any individual facility there is a point of minimum efficient scale beyond which further increases in patient load would entail increases in average cost per patient. Therefore, to reach more people, new facilities need to be developed, with appropriate staffing, support, and supplies. These facilities are likely to cover a smaller number of patients as they become more remote, so diseconomies are likely to develop related to the smaller-scale production. See Chapter 5 for a discussion of one promising policy response: increased delegation of tasks through task sharing with less specialized health care providers.

In looking at future numbers of HIV infections and numbers receiving treatment, the size of the population is important. Many African populations continue to grow, and population growth means that over time for a constant rate of infection, an increasing number of infections will be seen.

Cumulating Costs of Treatment

There are many models of the future course of the HIV/AIDS epidemic, which differ in their predictions according to the assumptions made. One model, produced for the *aids2031* project, predicts financing needs for both treatment and prevention for Africa through 2031 under four different scenarios: current trends, rapid scale-up of treatment and prevention, "hard choices," and "structural change" (an assumed change in behavior related to structural interventions [Gupta et al., 2008]).

According to this model, total required financing will be between $11 billion and $18 billion per year in 2020, depending on the scenario, as shown in Figure A-3. In this figure, *current trends* indicates that coverage of key interventions continues to expand to 2015 as it has in the past few years; *rapid scale-up* indicates that political will to achieve universal access is strong, and resource availability continues to grow rapidly; *hard choices* indicates that resources for HIV/AIDS programs are limited, so there is a focus on scaling up only the most cost-effective approaches for prevention; and *structural change* indicates a greater focus on structural change that can reduce vulnerability to HIV/AIDS and produce a more sustainable response (*aids2031* Costs and Financing Working Group, 2010).

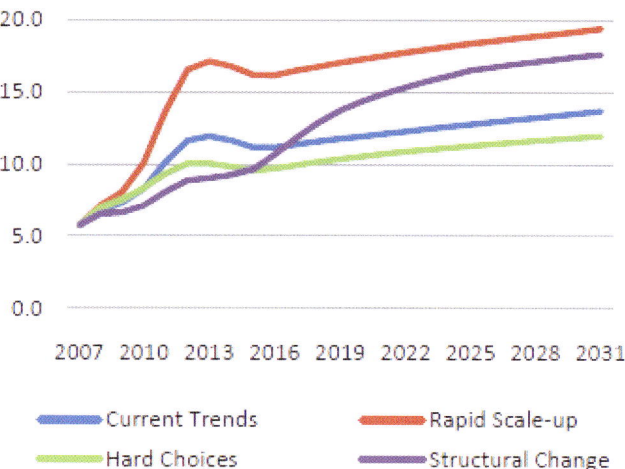

FIGURE A-3 One model predicts total financing needs of $11–18 billion in 2020, of which more than 25 percent would be for AIDS treatment.
SOURCE: *aids2031* Costs and Financing Working Group, 2010.

HIV/AIDS prevention costs are difficult to estimate because they are so elastic and because their efficacy is so poorly understood (Marseille et al., 2007). However, HIV/AIDS treatment costs are relatively easy to project, as discussed above and in Chapter 2.

It should be noted that treatment costs accumulate over time. Depending on policy choices currently available, the cumulated cost of HIV/AIDS treatment between 2010 and 2050 is likely to be between $200 billion and $800 billion (Figure A-4), assuming that incidence declines as shown in Panel b of Figures 2-3 and 2-4 in Chapter 2.

Nature of Treatment

In considering the future of the HIV/AIDS epidemic and associated patterns of treatment, the characteristics of the management of patients can be considered.

Syndromic Initiation

If HIV-positive individuals are diagnosed through testing for antibodies and the facilities for CD4 counts are unavailable, the only criterion for determining whether a patient should start therapy is symptoms. If diagnosis of HIV infection is timely, this reliance on symptoms will automatically reduce the average CD4 count at which patients start treatment and their chances of survival. Likewise,

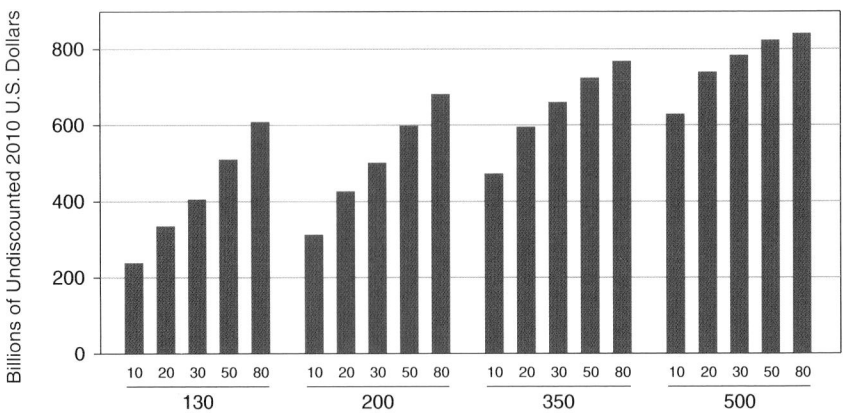

Uptake of Unmet Need 10%, 20%, 30%, 50%, and 80% and
Median CD4 Cell Count at Enrollment 130, 200, 350, and 500

FIGURE A-4 Cumulated cost of HIV/AIDS treatment in Africa through 2050 by the proportion of unmet need enrolled each year and the median CD4 cell count at enrollment. NOTE: Using the committee model, a bivariate sensitivity analysis comparing the influence of two parameters was used to show trade-offs, holding constant a set of epidemiological and cost assumptions as detailed in Annex A-1.
SOURCE: Committee projections using data from UNAIDS 2008.

where access to or uptake of counseling and testing is poor, people will be diagnosed as infected because of symptoms, and there will be a similar pattern of death. Using CD4 cell counts to determine the initiation of treatment is a simple and relatively inexpensive way of greatly improving the impact of treatment programs on years of life saved. However, questions arise of how frequently patients who are HIV-infected with a CD4 count above the initiation threshold should be monitored and how many tests should be done to confirm the accuracy of the CD4 measurement. As treatment coverage expanded, the initial goal was to find those in need of treatment and initiate them. However, as time progresses, those who did not initially need treatment will progress and become eligible. Either one can wait until people show symptoms, going back to the equivalent of syndromic initiation, or one can monitor their CD4 count over time.

Syndromic Management

A different set of questions arises about the management of those who have already been initiated on treatment. How frequently should they be seen? Should their CD4 count be monitored? What tests for toxicity of drugs are required?

And should measurements of viral load be made to identify successful viral suppression and failure? One approach is to manage syndromically; in a randomized controlled trial, such management was found to perform nearly as well as management with laboratory tests (Mugyenyi et al., 2010). However, failing to measure viral loads means that patients will have potentially high loads while they are exposed to antiretroviral drugs, providing selective pressure for the evolution of drug resistance (Gupta et al., 2009). The spread of resistant HIV would undermine the potential for successful treatment programs in the future (Blower et al., 2003).

Health Care Organization and Demands of Health Care Workers

The organization of health care can have an impact on the quality and accessibility of services, as well as their costs and feasibility. Who is legally and practically able to prescribe and administer antiretroviral drugs will depend upon the organization of health care in a country and the legal constraints on health care workers. A cascade model of care whereby patients with greater complications can be referred to secondary and tertiary services as required appears to be ideal, with less specialized health care workers maintaining patients on ART. Despite the potential for using workers with a range of skills, however, the demand for staff will be enormous if treatment is expanded to meet need. For example, in a

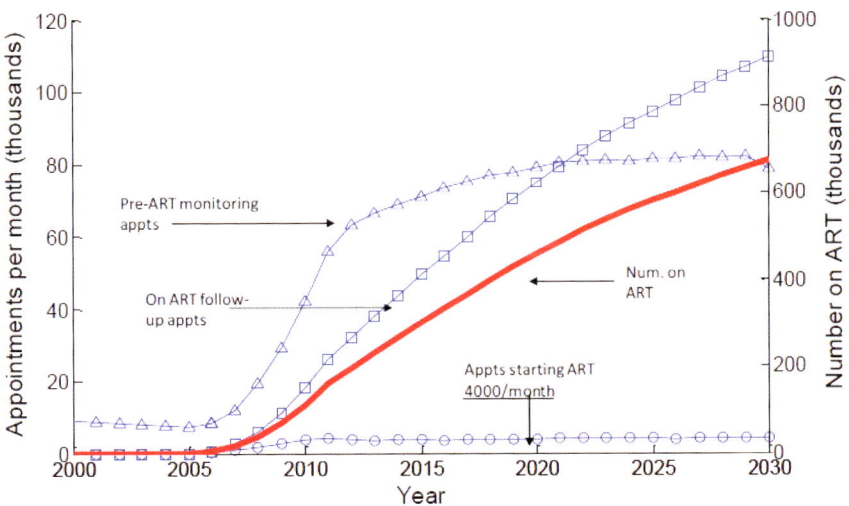

FIGURE A-5 Future treatment need and health system capacity in Zimbabwe.
NOTE: Universal access = 110,000 on treatment in 2010, 670,000 in 2030.
SOURCE: Hallett et al., in press.

modeling exercise focused on Zimbabwe, the number of appointments for monitoring patients over time can be predicted, revealing a large number of visits per health care worker per year. Chapter 5 examines the concept of task sharing, in which available personnel could redistribute the visits among a larger number of providers. Figure A-5 illustrates future treatment need and health system capacity in Zimbabwe.

REFERENCES

Aalen, O. O., V. T. Farewell, D. De Angelis, N. E. Day, and O. N. Gill. 1997. A Markov model for HIV disease progression including the effect of HIV diagnosis and treatment: Application to AIDS prediction in England and Wales. *Statistics in Medicine* 16(19):2191-2210.

Abbas, U. L., R. M. Anderson, and J. W. Mellors. 2006. Potential impact of antiretroviral therapy on HIV-1 transmission and AIDS mortality in resource-limited settings. *Journal of Acquired Immune Deficiency Syndromes* 41(5):632-641.

aids2031 Consortium. 2010. *aids2031: About*. http://www.aids2031.org/about (accessed October 21, 2010).

———. 2011. *AIDS: Taking a long-term view*. Upper Saddle River, NJ: Financial Times Science Press.

aids2031 Costs and Financing Working Group. 2010. *Costs and choices: Financing the long-term fight against AIDS*. Washington, DC: Results for Development Institute.

Baggaley, R. F., G. P. Garnett, and N. M. Ferguson. 2006. Modelling the impact of antiretroviral use in resource-poor settings. *PLoS Medicine* 3(4):e124.

Blower, S., E. Bodine, J. Kahn, and W. McFarland. 2005. The antiretroviral rollout and drug-resistant HIV in Africa: Insights from empirical data and theoretical models. *AIDS* 19(1):1-14.

Blower, S. M., A. N. Aschenbach, and J. O. Kahn. 2003. Predicting the transmission of drug-resistant HIV: Comparing theory with data. *The Lancet Infectious Diseases* 3(1):10-11.

Bollinger, L. A. 2008. How can we calculate the "E" in "CEA"? *AIDS* 22(Suppl. 1):S51-S57.

Bollinger, L., and J. Stover. 2010. *Estimating global resource needs for HIV/AIDS 2007-2031*. http://www.iom.edu/~/media/Files/Activity%20Files/Global/LongTermAIDS/2010-FEB-03/ Bollinger.pdf (accessed October 21, 2010).

Dodd, P. J., G. P. Garnett, and T. B. Hallett. 2010. Examining the promise of HIV elimination by "test and treat" in hyperendemic settings. *AIDS* 24(5):729-735.

Fenton, K. A., A. M. Johnson, S. McManus, and B. Erens. 2001. Measuring sexual behaviour: Methodological challenges in survey research. *Sexually Transmitted Infections* 77(2):84-92.

Garnett, G. P., J. M. Garcia-Calleja, T. Rehle, and S. Gregson. 2006. Behavioural data as an adjunct to HIV surveillance data. *Sexually Transmitted Infections* 82(Suppl. 1):i57-i62.

Granich, R. M., C. F. Gilks, C. Dye, K. M. De Cock, and B. G. Williams. 2009a. Universal voluntary HIV testing with immediate antiretroviral therapy as a strategy for elimination of HIV transmission: A mathematical model. *The Lancet* 373(9657):48-57.

———. 2009b. Universal voluntary HIV testing with immediate antiretroviral therapy as a strategy for elimination of HIV transmission: A mathematical model. *The Lancet* 373(9657):48-57.

Gupta, G. R., J. O. Parkhurst, J. A. Ogden, P. Aggleton, and A. Mahal. 2008. Structural approaches to HIV prevention. *The Lancet* 372(9640):764-775.

Gupta, R. K., A. Hill, A. W. Sawyer, A. Cozzi-Lepri, V. von Wyl, S. Yerly, V. D. Lima, H. F. Gunthard, C. Gilks, and D. Pillay. 2009. Virological monitoring and resistance to first-line highly active antiretroviral therapy in adults infected with HIV-1 treated under WHO guidelines: A systematic review and meta-analysis. *The Lancet Infectious Diseases* 9(7):409-417.

Hallett, T. B., S. Gregson, S. Dube, and G. P. Garnett. 2008. The impact of monitoring HIV patients prior to treatment in resource-poor settings: Insights from mathematical modelling. *PLoS Medicine* 5(3):e53.

Hallett, T. B., S. Dube, I. Cremin, B. Lopman, A. Mahomva, G. Ncube, O. Mugurungi, S. Gregson, and G. P. Garnett. 2009a. The role of testing and counseling for HIV prevention and care in the era of scaling-up antiretroviral therapy. *Epidemics* 1:77-82.

Hallett, T. B., S. Gregson, E. Gonese, O. Mugurungi, and G. P. Garnett. 2009b. Assessing evidence for behaviour change affecting the course of HIV epidemics: A new mathematical modelling approach and application to data from Zimbabwe. *Epidemics* 1:108-117.

Hallett, T. B., S. Gregson, S. Dube, E. S. Mapfeka, O. Mugurungi, and G. P. Garnett. In press. Estimating the resources required in the roll-out of universal access to antiretroviral therapy in Zimbabwe. *Sexually Transmitted Infections.*

Hecht, R., L. Bollinger, J. Stover, W. McGreevey, F. Muhib, C. E. Madavo, and D. de Ferranti. 2009. Critical choices in financing the response to the global HIV/AIDS pandemic. *Health Affairs* 28(6):1591-1605.

Hecht, R., J. Stover, L. Bollinger, F. Muhib, K. Case, and D. de Ferranti. 2010. Financing of HIV/AIDS programme scale up in low-income and middle-income countries, 2009-31. *The Lancet* 376(9748):1254-1260.

Johnson, L. 2010. *HIV/AIDS projections for South Africa.* Presentation to the IOM committee on envisioning a strategy to prepare for the long-term burden of HIV/AIDS: African needs and U.S. interests, Washington, DC, February 3, 2010.

Johnson, L. F., L. Alkema, and R. E. Dorrington. 2010. A Bayesian approach to uncertainty analysis of sexually transmitted infection models. *Sexually Transmitted Infections* 86(3):169-174.

Kimmel, A. D., S. J. Goldie, R. P. Walensky, E. Losina, M. C. Weinstein, A. D. Paltiel, H. Zhang, and K. A. Freedberg. 2005. Optimal frequency of CD4 cell count and HIV RNA monitoring prior to initiation of antiretroviral therapy in HIV-infected patients. *Antiviral Therapy* 10(1):41-52.

Levine, R. 2008. Healthy foreign policy: Bringing coherence to the global health agenda. In *The White House and the world: A global development agenda for the next U.S. president*, edited by N. Birdsall. Washington, DC: Center for Global Development.

Marseille, E., L. Dandona, N. Marshall, P. Gaist, S. Bautista-Arredondo, B. Rollins, S. Bertozzi, J. Coovadia, J. Saba, D. Lioznov, J.-A. Du Plessis, E. Krupitsky, N. Stanley, M. Over, A. Peryshkina, S. G. P. Kumar, S. Muyingo, C. Pitter, M. Lundberg, and J. Kahn. 2007. HIV prevention costs and program scale: Data from the PANCEA project in five low and middle-income countries. *BMC Health Services Research* 7(1):108.

Mngadi, S., N. Fraser, H. Mkhatshwa, T. Lapidos, T. Khumalo, S. Tsela, N. Nhlabatsi, and H. Odido. 2009. *Swaziland HIV prevention response and modes of transmission analysis.* Mbabane: National Emergency Response Council on HIV/AIDS, UNAIDS.

Mugyenyi, P., A. S. Walker, J. Hakim, P. Munderi, D. M. Gibb, C. Kityo, A. Reid, H. Grosskurth, J. H. Darbyshire, F. Ssali, D. Bray, E. Katabira, A. G. Babiker, C. F. Gilks, G. Kabuye, D. Nsibambi, R. Kasirye, E. Zalwango, M. Nakazibwe, B. Kikaire, G. Nassuna, R. Massa, K. Fadhiru, M. Namyalo, A. Zalwango, L. Generous, P. Khauka, N. Rutikarayo, W. Nakahima, A. Mugisha, J. Todd, J. Levin, S. Muyingo, A. Ruberantwari, P. Kaleebu, D. Yirrell, N. Ndembi, F. Lyagoba, P. Hughes, M. Aber, A. M. Lara, S. Foster, J. Amurwon, B. N. Wakholi, J. Whitworth, K. Wangati, B. Amuron, D. Kajungu, J. Nakiyingi, W. Omony, D. Tumukunde, T. Otim, J. Kabanda, H. Musana, J. Akao, H. Kyomugisha, A. Byamukama, J. Sabiiti, J. Komugyena, P. Wavamunno, S. Mukiibi, A. Drasiku, R. Byaruhanga, O. Labeja, P. Katundu, S. Tugume, P. Awio, A. Namazzi, G. T. Bakeinyaga, H. Katabira, D. Abaine, J. Tukamushaba, W. Anywar, W. Ojiambo, E. Angweng, S. Murungi, W. Haguma, S. Atwiine, J. Kigozi, L. Namale, A. Mukose, G. Mulindwa, D. Atwiine, A. Muhwezi, E. Nimwesiga, G. Barungi, J. Takubwa, D. Mwebesa, G. Kagina, M. Mulindwa, F. Ahimbisibwe, P. Mwesigwa, S. Akuma, C. Zawedde, D. Nyiraguhirwa, C. Tumusiime, L. Bagaya, W. Namara, J. Karungi, R. Kankunda, R. Enzama,

A. Latif, V. Robertson, E. Chidziva, R. Bulaya-Tembo, G. Musoro, F. Taziwa, C. Chimbetete, L. Chakonza, A. Mawora, C. Muvirimi, G. Tinago, P. Svovanapasis, M. Simango, O. Chirema, J. Machingura, S. Mutsai, M. Phiri, T. Bafana, M. Chirara, L. Muchabaiwa, M. Muzambi, J. Mutowo, T. Chivhunga, E. Chigwedere, M. Pascoe, C. Warambwa, E. Zengeza, F. Mapinge, S. Makota, A. Jamu, N. Ngorima, H. Chirairo, S. Chitsungo, J. Chimanzi, C. Maweni, R. Warara, M. Matongo, S. Mudzingwa, M. Jangano, K. Moyo, L. Vere, N. Mdege, I. Machingura, A. Ronald, A. Kambungu, F. Lutwama, I. Mambule, A. Nanfuka, J. Walusimbi, E. Nabankema, R. Nalumenya, T. Namuli, R. Kulume, I. Namata, L. Nyachwo, A. Florence, A. Kusiima, E. Lubwama, R. Nairuba, F. Oketta, E. Buluma, R. Waita, H. Ojiambo, F. Sadik, J. Wanyama, P. Nabongo, J. Oyugi, F. Sematala, A. Muganzi, C. Twijukye, H. Byakwaga, R. Ochai, D. Muhweezi, A. Coutinho, B. Etukoit, C. Gilks, K. Boocock, C. Puddephatt, C. Grundy, J. Bohannon, D. Winogron, A. Burke, A. Babiker, H. Wilkes, M. Rauchenberger, S. Sheehan, C. Spencer-Drake, K. Taylor, M. Spyer, A. Ferrier, B. Naidoo, D. Dunn, R. Goodall, L. Peto, R. Nanfuka, C. Mufuka-Kapuya, D. Pillay, A. McCormick, I. Weller, S. Bahendeka, M. Bassett, A. C. Wapakhabulo, B. Gazzard, C. Mapuchere, O. Mugurungi, C. Burke, S. Jones, C. Newland, G. Pearce, S. Rahim, J. Rooney, M. Smith, W. Snowden, J. M. Steens, A. Breckenridge, A. McLaren, C. Hill, J. Matenga, A. Pozniak, D. Serwadda, T. Peto, A. Palfreeman, and M. Borok. 2010. Routine versus clinically driven laboratory monitoring of HIV antiretroviral therapy in Africa (DART): A randomised non-inferiority trial. *The Lancet* 375(9709):123-131.

OGAC (Office of the Global AIDS Coordinator). 2010a. *Annual reports to Congress*. http://www. pepfar.gov/progress/index.htm (accessed June 3, 2010).

———. 2010b. *Operational plans*. http://www.pepfar.gov/about/c19388.htm (accessed June 3, 2010).

———. 2010c. *Report to Congress on costs of treatment in the President's Emergency Plan for AIDS Relief (PEPFAR)*. Washington, DC: PEPFAR.

Over, M. 2009. *AIDSCost computer program: Projecting future budgetary costs of AIDS treatment*. Center for Global Development. www.cgdev.org/files/1422227_file_AIDSCost_manual_FINAL.pdf (accessed October 29, 2010).

Over, M., and P. Piot. 1996. Human immunodeficiency virus infection and other sexually transmitted diseases in developing countries: Public health importance and priorities for resource allocation. *Journal of Infectious Diseases* 174(Suppl. 2):S162-S175.

Over, M., P. Heywood, J. Gold, I. Gupta, S. Hira, and E. Marseille. 2004. *HIV/AIDS treatment and prevention in India: Modeling the costs and consequences (health, nutrition, and population)*. Washington, DC: The World Bank.

Phillips, A. N., D. Pillay, A. H. Miners, D. E. Bennett, C. F. Gilks, and J. D. Lundgren. 2008. Outcomes from monitoring of patients on antiretroviral therapy in resource-limited settings with viral load, CD4 cell count, or clinical observation alone: A computer simulation model. *The Lancet* 371(9622):1443-1451.

Phillips, A. N., C. Gilks, and J. D. Lundgren. 2009. Cost-effectiveness of strategies for monitoring the response to antiretroviral therapy in resource-limited settings. *Archives of Internal Medicine* 169(9):904.

Slaymaker, E. 2004. A critique of international indicators of sexual risk behaviour. *Sexually Transmitted Infections* 80(Suppl. 2):ii13-ii21.

Stover, J., L. Bollinger, K. Cooper-Arnold, and The Futures Group International. 2003. *Goals model for estimating the effects of resource allocation decisions on the achievement of the goals of the HIV/AIDS Strategic Plan*. http://www.futuresinstitute.org/download/goals/Goals.pdf (accessed October 29, 2010).

Sweat, M., S. Gregorich, G. Sangiwa, C. Furlonge, D. Balmer, C. Kamenga, O. Grinstead, and T. Coates. 2000. Cost-effectiveness of voluntary HIV-1 counselling and testing in reducing sexual transmission of HIV-1 in Kenya and Tanzania. *The Lancet* 356(9224):113-121.

Todd, J., J. R. Glynn, M. Marston, T. Lutalo, S. Biraro, W. Mwita, V. Suriyanon, R. Rangsin, K. E. Nelson, P. Sonnenberg, D. Fitzgerald, E. Karita, and B. Zaba. 2007. Time from HIV seroconversion to death: A collaborative analysis of eight studies in six low and middle-income countries before highly active antiretroviral therapy. *AIDS* 21(Suppl. 6):S55-S63.

UNAIDS (The Joint United Nations Programme on HIV/AIDS). 2008. *Report on the global AIDS epidemic*. Geneva: UNAIDS.

———. 2010. *Fact sheet: Treatment 2.0*. Geneva: UNAIDS.

UNAIDS and WHO. 2009. *AIDS epidemic update: December 2009*. Geneva: UNAIDS.

UNAIDS/WHO/SACEMA Expert Group on Modelling the Impact and Cost of Male Circumcision for HIV Prevention. 2009. Male circumcision for HIV prevention in high HIV prevalence settings: What can mathematical modelling contribute to informed decision making? *PLoS Medicine* 6(9):e1000109.

Van Der Paal, L., L. A. Shafer, J. Todd, B. N. Mayanja, J. A. Whitworth, and H. Grosskurth. 2007. HIV-1 disease progression and mortality before the introduction of highly active antiretroviral therapy in rural Uganda. *AIDS* 21(Suppl. 6):S21-S29.

Velasco-Hernandez, J. X., H. B. Gershengorn, and S. M. Blower. 2002. Could widespread use of combination antiretroviral therapy eradicate HIV epidemics? *The Lancet Infectious Diseases* 2(8):487-493.

Venkatesh, K. K., G. de Bruyn, M. N. Lurie, L. Mohapi, P. Pronyk, M. Moshabela, E. Marinda, G. E. Gray, E. W. Triche, and N. A. Martinson. 2010. Decreased sexual risk behavior in the era of HAART among HIV-infected urban and rural South Africans attending primary care clinics. *Journal of Acquired Immune Deficiency Syndromes* 24(17):2687-96.

Wabwire-Mangen, F., M. Odiit, W. Kirungi, D. K. Kisitu, and J. O. Wanyama. 2009. *Uganda HIV modes of transmission and prevention response analysis*. Kampala: Uganda National AIDS Commission, UNAIDS.

Wagner, B., and S. Blower. 2009. Voluntary universal testing and treatment is unlikely to lead to HIV elimination: A modeling analysis. *Nature Precedings*. http://precedings.nature.com/documents/3917/version/1/files/npre20093917-1.pdf (accessed November 1, 2010).

White, R. G., K. K. Orroth, J. R. Glynn, E. E. Freeman, R. Bakker, J. D. Habbema, F. Terris-Prestholt, L. Kumaranayake, A. Buvé, and R. J. Hayes. 2008. Treating curable sexually transmitted infections to prevent HIV in Africa: Still an effective control strategy? *Journal of Acquired Immune Deficiency Syndromes* 47(3):346-353.

WHO (World Health Organization). 2010. *Towards universal access: Scaling up priority HIV/AIDS interventions in the health sector. Progress report 2010*. Geneva: WHO.

Williams, B. G., J. O. Lloyd-Smith, E. Gouws, C. Hankins, W. M. Getz, J. Hargrove, I. de Zoysa, C. Dye, and B. Auvert. 2006. The potential impact of male circumcision on HIV in sub-Saharan Africa. *PLoS Medicine* 3(7):e262.

ANNEX A-1
MODEL OF THE RELATIONSHIP
AMONG TREATMENT INITIATION,
COVERAGE, AND MORTALITY

A feature of a model with a user-selected target coverage rate is a pattern of rapid enrollment before the target rate is reached, followed by slow enrollment because the target has been reached. In such models, enrollment is largely unrelated to unmet need for treatment. An alternative approach is to specify the proportion of unmet need that the program absorbs every year, or the uptake rate, and allow this parameter to determine the growth of the coverage rate. The first approach—used, for example, in the *aids2031* model—allows enrollment to rapidly attain some target coverage rate regardless of the real absorptive capacity on the ground. The second approach—used, for example, in standard economic models of investment—is sometimes referred to as the "partial adjustment" model and captures the reality that programs typically cannot adjust by more than a percentage of unmet need in any given year. Under the first approach, a country is assumed to care about enrollment only until its coverage target is reached, whereas in the second, it is assumed to offer an equal chance at enrollment to those with unmet need in perpetuity. While real policy could follow either pattern, the partial adjustment approach better captures the policy reality of insufficient resources to enroll everyone who needs treatment by any given definition.

Assuming a constant rate of people becoming newly in need of treatment, b, and the death rate of those in need, α, and those on treatment, μ, we can calculate the relationship between the fraction of those newly in need starting treatment immediately, ϕ; the rate of those in need starting treatment, γ; and the patterns of treatment coverage and mortality. Where X is the number in need but not yet on treatment and Y is the number on treatment, the rate of change of these numbers is given by the ordinary differential equations

$$\frac{dX}{dt} = (1-\varphi)b - \gamma X - \alpha X$$

$$\frac{dY}{dt} = \varphi b + \gamma X - \mu Y$$

These equations have the equilibrium solution:

$$X^* = \frac{(1-\varphi)b}{(\gamma+\alpha)}; Y^* = \frac{\left[\varphi b + \gamma \frac{(1-\varphi b)}{(\gamma+\alpha)}\right]}{\mu}$$

If the coverage of treatment is defined as the proportion in need, coverage at equilibrium is:

$$C = \frac{Y^*}{(X^*+Y^*)} = \frac{\dfrac{\left[\varphi + \gamma\dfrac{(1-\varphi)}{(\gamma+\alpha)}\right]}{\mu}}{\left\{\dfrac{(1-\varphi)}{(\gamma+\alpha)} + \dfrac{\left[\varphi + \gamma\dfrac{(1-\varphi)}{(\gamma+\alpha)}\right]}{\mu}\right\}}$$

The number of deaths is simply $\alpha X + \mu Y$.

For given rates of HIV incidence and treatment initiation, an HIV epidemic will approach a long-run equilibrium coverage rate, which for high incidence and low treatment initiation will be substantially less than universal coverage.

ANNEX A-2
WHAT DRIVES THE DIFFERENCES
AMONG PROJECTIONS

Various models include different levels of detail. The models of Blower assume a homogeneous population with respect to risk behavior, which allows a wider spread of HIV with a lower reproductive number than would be the case with a model including heterogeneity in risk (Blower et al., 2003, 2005). The model of Granich is also homogeneous with respect to risk, but it assumes that the incidence of infection is inversely proportional to prevalence, which allows prevalence to saturate and stabilize despite a higher basic reproductive number (Granich et al., 2009b). The models of Baggaley, Phillips, and Johnson include distributions of risk across the population (Baggaley et al., 2006; Johnson et al., 2010; Phillips et al., 2008). This heterogeneity in risk is observed in reported behavioral data, but the fine details are less certain. These models of Blower, Granich, Baggaley, Phillips, and Johnson have been used to explore a number of HIV/AIDS prevention interventions, including the impact of treatments for sexually transmitted infections (STIs) (Over and Piot, 1996; White et al., 2008), of adult male circumcision (UNAIDS/WHO/SACEMA Expert Group on Modelling the Impact and Cost of Male Circumcision for HIV Prevention, 2009; Williams et al., 2006), of counseling and testing (Hallett et al., 2009a), and of treatment (Abbas et al., 2006; Baggaley et al., 2006; Dodd et al., 2010; Velasco-Hernandez et al., 2002). The effect size of interventions will depend greatly on how resilient the spread of the virus is, which in turn depends on the importance assumed in the model for a high-risk group driving the epidemic. In addition, the frequency of unprotected sex and the pattern of mixing specific to different activity groups have an impact on model results. Other differences in models result from different definitions of coverage and the long-term impact of treatment. For example, the Goals model used by *aids2031* (Bollinger and Stover, 2010; Hecht et al., 2010; Stover et al., 2003) and the AIDSCost model used by the committee (Over, 2009) both assume that after the first year, treatment failure occurs at a constant rate. This is a more pessimistic assumption than would be expected from the impact of treatment in developing countries.

Models with detailed patterns of risk behavior require many input parameters that can be estimated from local studies of behavior or from a fit between the observed epidemiology of HIV and the model outputs. Unfortunately, models that include a description of the range of behavioral interactions within populations will be overspecified, with multiple parameter sets being able to generate the observed epidemics. To an extent, this issue is being addressed in the development of models of HIV transmission (Hallett et al., 2009b; Johnson et al., 2010) in which multiple datasets are being combined for analysis. However, the detailed work required for predictions in one location does not allow for a complete picture of the HIV/AIDS epidemic in Africa. In exercises across a wide range of countries, simpler methods have been applied, either using one "reasonable" parameter set (Hecht et al., 2010) or using estimated incidence at a recent time point as an input (Levine, 2008). The approach adopted by the committee in its model is to assume that interventions could achieve progressive reductions in incidence if sufficient incentives were provided (Over, 2009). This assumption allows the benefits of reduced incidence to be calculated without defining exactly how it is to be achieved.

To calculate the fraction of those infected needing treatment, a rate of progression to treatment need is applied. Of those needing treatment, a fraction receive it (this is the rate of treatment coverage per year). After 1 year, a fraction fail treatment and either die or are placed on second-line treatment, for which there is a further rate of treatment failure that is assumed to lead to death.

Estimating the future incidence of HIV based on incidence in a baseline year provides a basis for calculations that take account of future changes in coverage of treatment and prevention interventions. However, to represent the influence of a "core group" that has a high rate of HIV acquisition and transmission and therefore drives the epidemiology of infection, it is necessary to limit the fraction of the population susceptible to infection, k. A baseline incidence rate, IR_0, is assigned to the year 2007—$IR_0 = IR_{2007}$—which is an input variable that can be derived from the absolute incidence, AI_0, in each country.

Since the absolute incidence is a function of the incidence rate and the fraction of the population to which it is applied, three different approaches are possible: to hold the incidence rate constant across countries, to hold a fraction of the population at risk constant across countries, or to vary both across countries. To reflect the very different prevalences across Africa, which presumably reflect the fraction of the population engaging in risk behaviors, country-specific fractions at risk, k, are estimated from a constant incidence rate:

$$k = \frac{AI_0 + IR_0 H_0}{IR_0 P_{15\ 0}^{69}}$$

where H_0 is the number HIV-infected, and $P_{15\ 0}^{69}$ is the total population aged 15–64. IR_0 is an external variable. A high value—for example, 0.2—would generate a low value of k relative to the prevalence in year zero and make HIV difficult to control compared with a high value of IR_0—for example, 0.01—which would generate a high value of k.

For future years, the above equation is rearranged to calculate the absolute number of new infections, which is a function of the incidence rate:

$$AI_t = IR_t P_{15\ t}^{69} (k[1 + \Delta.\theta_t] - \text{Prev}_t$$

The prevalence at time t, $Prev_t$, is the number infected, H_t, divided by the population size, $P_{15\ t}^{69}$. The proportion of those HIV-infected who are on treatment, θ_t, is assumed to influence the fraction of the population at risk through disinhibition, which is determined by the parameter Δ. If this value is negative, it is assumed that treatment acts to reduce the fraction of the population engaging in risk behaviors. The incidence rate is a function of changes in the prevalence of infection (i.e., the pool of infectious contacts within the population); prevention interventions that reduce susceptibility to infection and risk behaviors; and the proportion of those infectious with a reduced viraemia due to treatment relative to the baseline proportion treated:

$$IR_t = IR_0 \frac{Prev_t \tau_t}{Prev_0 \tau_o (1 - c_t.m.\varepsilon)(1-\omega_t)(1-\delta\theta_t)}$$

where the impact of treatment on infection, τ_t, is given by $\tau_t = (1 - f.g.\theta_t)$, where θ_t is the proportion of those infected treated, f is the fraction of infection that occurs after the initial primary viraemia, and g is the proportional reduction in transmissibility of those on treatment. The fraction of adult men circumcised is given by c, m is the proportion of adults that are men, and ε is the reduced susceptibility associated with circumcision. The parameter ω_t represents prevention effort. Both the proportion circumcised and effort are externally input functions of time with a linear increase to a maximum value.

2:15 pm–2:30 pm	Research/Academic Perspective **Neal Nathanson,** University of Pennsylvania
2:30 pm–2:45 pm	Security Perspective **Steve Morrison**, Center for Strategic and International Studies
2:45 pm–3:15 pm	Moderated Question and Answer Session
3:15 pm–3:25 pm	Break

SESSION 4—OPEN

STATEMENT OF TASK #4: ORGANIZATIONAL STRATEGIES TO BUILD LONG-TERM CAPACITY

Statement of Task #4: What should be the strategies for the United States to develop now in order to ensure domestic and international capacities for highly effective HIV prevention, treatment, and care efforts in the 2018–2023 time frame? What structures, systems, and professions would be necessary to implement these strategies?

Moderators: Francis Omaswa, Carmen Portillo, and Marla Salmon

3:25 pm–3:40 pm	UNAIDS Strategy **David Wilson**, UNAIDS
3:40 pm–3:55 pm	PEPFAR Strategy **Joan Holloway,** Office of the U.S. Global AIDS Coordinator
3:55 pm–4:10 pm	U.S. State Department Strategy **Sue K. Brown**, State Department
4:10 pm–4:25 pm	World Bank Strategy **David Wilson**, World Bank
4:25 pm–5:00 pm	Moderated Question and Answer Session
5:00 pm	Adjourn for the Day

THURSDAY, FEBRUARY 4, 2010
Room 206

SESSION 5 AND 6—CLOSED

REACTIONS TO PRESENTATIONS;
DRAFT CONCLUSIONS AND RECOMMENDATIONS

SESSION 7—OPEN

REVISITING STATEMENT OF TASK #4:
SPECIFIC STRATEGIES TO BUILD LONG-TERM CAPACITY

Statement of Task #4: What should be the strategies for the United States
to develop now in order to ensure domestic and international capacities for
highly effective HIV prevention, treatment, and care efforts in the 2018–2023
time frame? What structures, systems, and professions would be necessary to
implement these strategies?

Moderators: Francis Omaswa, Carmen Portillo, and Marla Salmon

1:15 pm–1:25 pm	Educational Collaboratives **Kathy Cahill,** Cahill, Davila and Associates
1:25 pm–1:35 pm	Informatics **Patti Abbott,** Johns Hopkins University
1:35 pm–1:45 pm	Academic Partnership, Electronic Health Records **Robert Einterz,** Indiana University
1:45 pm–1:55 pm	Strategies for NGOs to Build HIV/AIDS Capacity in Africa **Leslie Mancuso,** JHPIEGO
1:55 pm–2:45 pm	Moderated Question and Answer Session

1:45 pm–2:45 pm	Moderated Panel Discussion

2:45 pm–3:00 pm	Break

SESSION 4:
ETHICAL IMPLICATIONS OF THE HIV/AIDS EPIDEMIC

Session Moderator: **Ames Dhai**, Committee Member

3:00 pm–3:20 pm	Building African Capacity to Assure Long-Term Procedural Justice in Situations of Scarce Resource Allocation **Mark Heywood**, AIDS Law Project

3:20 pm–3:40 pm	Global Responsibilities: African Response **Elizabeth Bukusi,** Kenya Medical Research Institute

3:40 pm–4:00 pm	Global Responsibilities: Western Response **Devi Sridhar**, Oxford University

4:00 pm–5:00 pm	Moderated Panel Discussion

5:00 pm–7:00 pm	Reception for Committee, Speakers, and All Workshop Attendees

TUESDAY, APRIL 13, 2010

9:00 am–9:10 am	Welcome and Recap of Day 1 **Tom Quinn** and **David Serwadda**, Committee Co-Chairs

SESSION 5: BUILDING AFRICAN CAPACITY FOR HIV/AIDS

Session Moderator: **Carmen Portillo**, Committee Member

9:10 am–9:25 am	The Role of NGOs in Building Capacity for HIV/AIDS **Paula Akugizibwe**, AIDS & Rights Alliance for Southern Africa

9:25 am–9:40 am   The Role of the Private Sector in Building Capacity for
                       HIV/AIDS
                       Jenni Gillies, SABMiller

9:40 am–9:55 am   The Role of Faith-Based Organizations in Building
                       Capacity for HIV/AIDS
                       Ruth Stark, Catholic Relief Services

9:55 am–10:10 am   The Role of Professional Associations in Building
                       Capacity for HIV/AIDS
                       Leana Uys, International Council of Nurses

10:10 am–11:10 am   Moderated Panel Discussion

11:10 am–11:25 am   Break

SESSION 6: BUILDING AFRICAN ACADEMIC
AND RESEARCH CAPACITY IN HIV/AIDS

Session Moderator: **Peter Ndumbe**, Committee Member

11:25 am–11:40 am   The Role of Academia in Building Capacity for HIV/
                       AIDS
                       Umesh Lalloo, Nelson R. Mandela School of Medicine

11:40 am–11:55 am   Medical Education Partnership Initiative and the Role
                       of Fogarty-funded Initiatives in Building Capacity for
                       HIV/AIDS
                       Michael Johnson, U.S. National Institutes of Health,
                       Fogarty Center

11:55 am–12:10 pm   The Role of Science Academies in Building Capacity
                       for HIV/AIDS
                       Tony Mbewu, Global Forum for Health Research,
                       Academy of Science of South Africa (ASSAf)

12:10 pm–12:25 pm   Building African Research and Treatment Capacity
                       James Hakim, University of Zimbabwe

12:25 pm–1:15 pm   Moderated Panel Discussion

1:15 pm–2:15 pm   Lunch

SESSION 7: TWINNING PARTNERSHIPS TO BUILD LONG-TERM CAPACITY FOR HIV/AIDS

Session Moderator: **Francis Omaswa**, Committee Member

2:15 pm–2:30 pm	University Partnerships **Sylvester Kimaiyo**, Academic Model Providing Access to Healthcare
2:30 pm–2:45 pm	Military Partnerships **Darrell Singer**, U.S. Department of Defense HIV Program, Nigeria
2:45 pm–3:00 pm	South–South Partnerships and Regional Strategies **Quarraisha Abdool Karim**, Centre for AIDS Programme of Research, South Africa
3:00 pm–3:15 pm	Laboratory Systems Strengthening Initiative **Danni Ramduth**, Becton, Dickinson and Company
3:15 pm–4:15 pm	Moderated Panel Discussion
4:15 pm–5:00 pm	Open Forum for Discussion, Closing Remarks, and Wrap-up **Tom Quinn and David Serwadda**, Committee Co-Chairs
5:00 pm	Adjourn

Appendix D

Committee Member Biographical Sketches

Thomas C. Quinn, M.D., M.Sc. (Co-Chair), is associate director for international research and head of the section on International HIV/AIDS Research in the Laboratory of Immunoregulation at the National Institute of Allergy and Infectious Diseases. Dr. Quinn is also director of the Johns Hopkins Center for Global Health, facilitating international research at the allied health institutions of The Johns Hopkins University. He is a professor of medicine and pathology in the Johns Hopkins School of Medicine and holds adjunct appointments in the Departments of International Health, Epidemiology, and Molecular Microbiology and Immunology in the Johns Hopkins Bloomberg School of Public Health. Dr. Quinn is board certified in internal medicine and infectious diseases and is on the clinical staff of Johns Hopkins Hospital and the National Institutes of Health (NIH) Clinical Center. His investigations have addressed the epidemiologic, virologic, and immunologic features of HIV infection in Africa, the Caribbean, South America, and Asia. In 1983, he led the first group of scientists to Haiti and central Africa to determine the extent of HIV within those countries. In 1984, he helped establish an interagency project called "Project SIDA" in Kinshasa, Zaire, which was the largest AIDS investigative project in sub-Saharan Africa. Since then he has generated numerous global initiatives and research programs in 28 countries. Dr. Quinn and his colleagues in Rakai, Uganda, demonstrated that HIV viral load was the single most important predictor of HIV perinatal and sexual transmission, correlating this with timing of infection and natural history. In 2004, Dr. Quinn was elected to the Institute of Medicine (IOM). He is a fellow of the Infectious Disease Society of America, a fellow of the American Association for the Advancement of Science, a member of the American Association of Physicians, and a member of the American Society for Clinical Investigation. He is a founding member of the Academic Alliance for AIDS Care and Prevention in Africa and helped design the Infectious Diseases Institute of Makerere University School of Medicine, where he also holds an adjunct appointment in medicine. Dr. Quinn is the recipient of multiple awards and honors and is the author of more than 800 publications on HIV, sexually transmitted diseases (STDs), and infectious diseases.

David Serwadda, M.B.Ch.B., M.Med, M.Sc., M.P.H. (Co-Chair), is an infectious disease epidemiologist and professor and former dean of the School of Public Health at Makerere University in Kampala. He received his M.B.Ch.B., and M.Med (internal medicine) from Makerere University and an M.P.H. from the Johns Hopkins Bloomberg School of Public Health. Dr. Serwadda was among the first researchers to report on the presence of HIV/AIDS in Uganda (*Lancet*, 1985) and has worked continuously on research related to the evaluation of population-based HIV interventions to reduce transmission since the mid-1980s. He has been a senior investigator in the Rakai Health Science Program since its inception in 1988 and is the Ugandan principal investigator on the ongoing NIH-funded Trial of Male Circumcision for HIV Prevention. He has been instrumental in the scientific design and management of the project and has served as a critical liaison among the project; the local community; Ugandan political and policy decision makers; the Ugandan Ministry of Health; and international agencies including the Joint United Nations Programme on HIV/AIDS (UNAIDS), the World Health Organization (WHO), and the World Bank.

Salim S. Abdool Karim, M.B.Ch.B., Ph.D., is an infectious diseases epidemiologist and pro vice-chancellor (research) at the University of KwaZulu-Natal in Durban. He is director of the Centre for the AIDS Program of Research in South Africa (CAPRISA). He is also professor of clinical epidemiology at Columbia University and adjunct professor of medicine at Cornell University. Dr. Abdool Karim's research focuses on HIV epidemiology, HIV prevention through microbicides and vaccines, and treatment of HIV–TB coinfection. He was coprincipal investigator for the landmark CAPRISA 004 trial, which provided proof-of-concept that a microbicide prevents HIV infection. He is also coinventor of two HIV vaccine-related patents and has focused on the critical design challenges in HIV vaccine trials. His research on HIV–TB treatment has shaped the current therapeutic approach to treating coinfected patients and led to the 2009 revision of the WHO guidelines for treatment of HIV and TB coinfection. Dr. Abdool Karim serves on the Global HIV Vaccine Enterprise; the Scientific Advisory Board of the International AIDS Vaccine Initiative; the Gates Foundation's Global HIV Prevention Working Group; the UNAIDS Prevention Reference Group; and the WHO Expert Advisory Panel on Sexually Transmitted Infections, including HIV. He is chair of the WHO Scientific and Technical Advisory Group for Reproductive Health. He is also a member of the Academy of Science of South Africa and a fellow of the South African Royal Society of Science.

Jennifer G. Cooke, M.A., is director of the Center for Strategic and International Studies (CSIS) Africa Program, which she joined in 2000. She works on a range of U.S.–Africa policy issues, including security, health, conflict, and democratization. She has written numerous reports, articles, and commentaries for a range of U.S. and international publications. With J. Stephen Morrison, she is coeditor of *U.S. Africa Policy Beyond the Bush Administration: Critical Challenges for the Obama Administration* (CSIS, 2009), as well as a previous volume titled *Africa Policy in the Clinton Years: Critical Choices for the Bush Administration* (CSIS, 2001). Previously, she worked for the House Foreign Affairs Subcommittee on Africa, as well as for the National Academy of Sciences' Office of News and Public Information and Committee on Human Rights. Ms. Cooke has lived in Côte d'Ivoire and the Central Africa Republic. She earned an M.A. in African studies and international economics from the Johns Hopkins School of Advanced International Studies and a B.A. in government from Harvard University.

Amaboo (Ames) Dhai, M.B.Ch.B., FCOG, LLM, is director of the Steve Biko Centre for Bioethics at the University of the Witwatersrand Medical School. She started her career as a medical doctor when she obtained an M.B.Ch.B. through the University of Natal. She thereafter specialized as an obstetrician/gynecologist through the Colleges of Medicine, South Africa. She subsequently obtained an LLM through the Law School of the University of Natal and a diploma in international research ethics at the University of Cape Town. She was appointed head of bioethics, medical law, and research ethics at the Nelson R. Mandela School of Medicine in 2004, and in January 2006 took on the position of head of bioethics at the University of the Witwatersrand Medical School. Dr. Dhai's special interest is research ethics. She served as chair of the Research Ethics Committee of the University of KwaZulu-Natal for 2 years and as a member of the Interim National Ministerial Research Ethics Committee during 2002–2005, and in 2006 she was appointed deputy chair of the National Health Research Ethics Council. Currently, she serves on the Medical Research Council (MRC) Ethics Committee. She established and chairs the Hospice Palliative Care of South Africa Research Ethics Committee and is cochair of the Wits Human Research Ethics Committee (Medical). She also serves on the Medical and Dental Board of the Health Professions Council of South Africa and the Council of the Colleges of Obstetricians and Gynecologists of South Africa and is a member of the Human Rights, Ethics and Professional Development Committee of the Health Professions Council and the Human Rights and Ethics Committee of the South African Medical Association. Dr. Dhai was recently appointed to the National Biotechnology Advisory Committee, which has been tasked to offer specialist advice to the Minister of Science and Technology. Her publications address mainly issues of bioethics and medical law. She is editor-in-chief of the *South African Journal of Bioethics and Law*.

Geoffrey P. Garnett, Ph.D., is professor of microparasite epidemiology in the Department of Infectious Disease Epidemiology and director of a masters program in epidemiology at the Imperial College London. He holds a Ph.D. in pure science from the University of Sheffield, where he studied the transmission dynamics of varicella-zoster virus. He has worked on the epidemiology of STDs, including HIV, since 1990, with an interest in mathematical models of the clinical course of infections, patterns of sexual behavior, and patterns of infection. He has collaborated on community randomized trials of HIV and STD interventions and developed observational methods for tracking changes in HIV risk. He has developed models to explore the impact of prevention and treatment interventions and serves as chair of the UNAIDS Reference Group on Estimates, Models, and Projections.

Peter Ndumbe, M.D., has served as dean of the Faculty of Health Sciences of the University of Buea in Cameroon since December 2006. Previously he was dean of the Faculty of Medicine and Biomedical Sciences of the University of Yaoundé from January 1999 to December 2006. He is professor of virus immunology and director of the Centre for the Study and Control of Communicable Diseases at the University of Yaoundé. Professor Ndumbe is vice chair of the Scientific Committee of the Chantal Biya International Research Centre on HIV/AIDS and related diseases, created by the First Lady of Cameroon. He is also 2nd vice chair of the Cameroon Academy of Sciences. Prior to becoming dean, Professor Ndumbe was deputy director general of the Institute of Medical Research and Studies on Medicinal Plants in Cameroon. He was the founding director of Cam-diagnostix, a center for the production of diagnostic kits for the detection of HIV and hepatitis B. He has also served as chair of the National AIDS Commission of Cameroon. In WHO, Professor Ndumbe is a member of several committees, serving among other functions as chair of the Scientific and Technical Advisory Committee of the Tropical Diseases Research program and chair of the Advisory Committee on Research of the Initiative for Vaccine Research. His research interests are in HIV, STDs, vaccine-preventable diseases, and health systems for the delivery of interventions.

Francis Omaswa, M.D., is executive director of the African Center for Global Health and Social Transformation (ACHEST), a think tank that aspires to stimulate the building of transformational African capacity for leadership in health and is based in Kampala, Uganda. Until May 2008, he was founding executive director of the Global Health Workforce Alliance (GHWA), whose secretariat is provided by WHO headquarters in Geneva. There he coordinated the design and adoption of the Kampala Declaration and Agenda for Global Action on the

Health Workforce that now guides the global response to the health workforce crisis. He was director general of health services in the Ministry of Health in Uganda, during which time he coordinated major reforms in the health sector and was instrumental in drafting the African Union's Abuja Declaration on HIV/AIDS and was a member of the task forces that developed its implementation and monitoring framework. He was lead consultant in the development of the African Union HIV/AIDS Strategy in 2004. Dr. Omaswa has been active in international health, serving as chair/vice chair of the STOP TB Partnership and chair of the Global Fund Portfolio and Procurement Committee; he is currently chair of the Global Alliance for Vaccines and Immunisation (GAVI) Independent Review Committee and the sub-Saharan African Medical Schools Study. He is a graduate of Makerere University Medical School, Kampala, Uganda. He has held teaching appointments at Makerere University and Nairobi University, is a senior associate at the Johns Hopkins Bloomberg School of Public Health, and is chancellor of Busitema University in Uganda.

Mead Over, Ph.D., is a senior fellow at the Center for Global Development (CGD), conducting research on the economics of efficient, effective, and cost-effective health interventions in developing countries. Holding a Ph.D. from the University of Wisconsin, Dr. Over taught econometrics and health economics for 11 years at Williams College and then at Boston University, leaving for The World Bank in 1986 with the rank of associate professor. Much of his work since 1987, for 20 years at The World Bank and now at the CGD, is on the economics of the HIV/AIDS epidemic. After working on the economic impact of the epidemic and on cost-effective interventions, he coauthored the Bank's first comprehensive treatment of the economics of AIDS—the book *Confronting AIDS: Public Priorities for a Global Epidemic* (1997, 1999). Dr. Over's most recent book is entitled *The Economics of Effective AIDS Treatment: Evaluating Policy Options for Thailand* (2006). His forthcoming book from the CGD is entitled *Achieving the AIDS Transition: Preventing Infections to Sustain Treatment.* Papers he has published examine the economics of preventing and of treating malaria. He is currently working on the efficiency of AIDS service delivery in poor countries.

Carmen Portillo, R.N., Ph.D., FAAN, is codirector of a Health Resources and Services Administration (HRSA)-sponsored nurse capacity development and health systems strengthening twinning project funded through the American International Health Alliance. Since 2006, this project has collaborated with the School of Nursing, Muhimbili University of Health and Allied Sciences, and the Ministry of Health, Nursing Unit, in Dar es Salaam, Tanzania. Dr. Portillo is professor and chair of the Department of Community Health Systems, School of Nursing, at the University of California, San Francisco (SON, UCSF). She is currently director of the HIV Advanced Practice Nurse Education Program and codirector of the International Center for HIV/AIDS Research and Clinical

Training in Nursing at SON, UCSF, and for the last 9 years has been a senior advisory nurse for the International Training and Education Center for Health (I-TECH). Her research focuses on HIV/AIDS, particularly in women; adherence issues and stigma; and Hispanic health issues. She is a member of the Association of Nurses in AIDS Care and a fellow in the American Academy of Nursing.

Jessica E. Price, Ph.D., has been engaged in designing, implementing, and documenting outcomes of HIV interventions in sub-Saharan Africa since 1989. Over the years, working closely with African government, academic, private-sector, and civil society institutions, Dr. Price has led large technical assistance programs aimed at strategically introducing and scaling up new services and approaches in HIV prevention, care, and treatment, as well as at contributing to broader needs in national health sector plans and strategies. Dr. Price received her Ph.D. in cultural anthropology from Case Western Reserve University in 2002, with a specialization in health and illness. At present, she is Family Health International's (FHI's) technical director for Africa. She has also served as FHI country director in Rwanda and Kenya, performed several short-term consultancies to support national health programs in Africa, and held faculty positions in anthropology in the United States.

Marla Salmon, Sc.D., R.N., FAAN, is Robert G. and Jean A. Reid Dean in Nursing and professor of psychosocial and community health at the University of Washington School of Nursing, and professor of global health in the University's School of Public Health. Dr. Salmon was previously dean and professor at Emory University School of Nursing, where she was also founding director of the Lillian Carter Center for International Nursing. She has held academic leadership positions in nursing and public health at the University of Pennsylvania, the University of North Carolina, and the University of Minnesota. Dr. Salmon's scholarship and policy leadership have focused on national and international health workforce development, with a particular emphasis on policy and capacity building. She served as director of the Division of Nursing for the U.S. Department of Health and Human Services, where she also chaired the National Advisory Council for Nurse Education and Practice and served on the White House Taskforce on Healthcare Reform. She has served as a consultant and senior advisor to numerous governments and international organizations, including WHO, Commonwealth, the Pan American Health Organization, and Caribbean Community. Dr. Salmon has served on numerous boards and advisory groups, including her current membership on The Robert Wood Johnson Foundation Board of Trustees, the NIH National Advisory Council for Nursing Research, the Institute for the International Education of Students (IES), and the Joint Commission on Accreditation of Healthcare Organizations' Nursing Advisory Council. She is a member of the IOM and a fellow of the American Academy of Nursing. The recipient of numerous honors and recognitions for leadership in nursing and public health, Dr. Salmon holds a doctor of science degree from the Johns Hopkins University and a BSN, BA in political science and an MSN from the University of Portland (Oregon), and was a Fulbright Scholar in Germany. She holds three honorary degrees.

Scholar-in-Residence

Elena O. Nightingale, M.D., Ph.D., is a scholar-in-residence at the IOM and adjunct professor of pediatrics at both Georgetown University Medical Center and George Washington University Medical Center. Previously, she was special advisor to the president and senior program officer at Carnegie Corporation of New York and lecturer in social medicine at Harvard University. She retired from both positions at the end of 1994. Dr. Nightingale earned an A.B. degree in zoology, summa cum laude, from Barnard College of Columbia University; a Ph.D. in microbial genetics from the Rockefeller University; and an M.D. from New York University School of Medicine. With Eric Stover, she coedited *The Breaking of Bodies and Minds: Torture, Psychiatric Abuse and the Health Professions*, published in 1985, one of the earliest efforts to discuss this topic. She is also coeditor of *Promoting the Health of Adolescents: New Directions for the 21st Century* and *Prenatal Screening, Policies, and Values: The Example of Neural Tube Defects*. She coauthored *Before Birth: Prenatal Testing for Genetic Disease* and has authored numerous book chapters and articles on microbial genetics, child and adolescent health, health promotion and disease prevention, health policy, and human rights. Dr. Nightingale continues to be active in the protection of human rights, particularly those of children, and serves on the Advisory Committee of the Children's Rights Division of Human Rights Watch. She is a member of the IOM and of the IOM Roundtable on Health Disparities and the Report Review Committee of the National Academies. In 2006, she received the Walsh McDermott medal in recognition of her distinguished service to the IOM and the National Academies. In 2008, in recognition of extraordinary service, she was designated a lifetime national associate of the National Research Council of the National Academies.

Consultants

Robert Black, M.D., M.P.H., is chair of the Department of International Health and Edgar Berman Professor in International Health, as well as director of the Institute for International Programs, at the Johns Hopkins Bloomberg School of Public Health. Dr. Black is trained in medicine, infectious diseases, and epidemiology. He has served as a medical epidemiologist at the U.S. Centers for Disease Control and Prevention and worked at institutions in Bangladesh and Peru on research related to childhood infectious diseases and nutritional problems. Dr. Black's current research includes field trials of vaccines, micronutrients, and other nutritional interventions; effectiveness studies of health programs; and evaluation of preventive and curative health service programs in low- and middle-income countries. His other interests are related to the use of evidence in policy and programs, including estimates of burden of disease and the development of research capacity. As a member of the IOM and advisory bodies of WHO, the International Vaccine Institute, and other international organizations, he assists with the development of policies intended to improve child health. He chairs the Child Health Epidemiology Reference Group and the Child Health and Nutrition Research Initiative. He currently is involved in projects in Bangladesh, Ghana, India, Malawi, Mali, Peru, Tanzania, and Zanzibar. Dr. Black has authored more than 450 scientific journal publications and is coeditor of the textbook *International Public Health*. He has served on four committees and the Board on International Health (now Global Health) of the IOM.

Lawrence Gostin, J.D., is an internationally acclaimed scholar. He is Linda D. and Timothy J. O'Neill Professor of Global Health Law at the Georgetown University Law Center, where he directs the O'Neill Institute for National and Global Health Law. He served as associate dean for research at Georgetown Law until 2008. He is also professor of public health at the Johns Hopkins and Georgetown Universities—a Collaborating Center of WHO and the Centers for Disease Control and Prevention. He is visiting professor of public health (Faculty of Medical Sciences) and research fellow (Centre for Socio-Legal Studies) at Oxford University. Prof. Gostin is health law and ethics editor, contributing writer, and columnist for the *Journal of the American Medical Association*. In 2007, the director general of WHO appointed him to the International Health Regulations (IHR) Roster of Experts and the Expert Advisory Panel on Mental Health. Prof. Gostin holds three honorary degrees. An elected lifetime Member of the IOM, he serves on the Board on Health Sciences Policy and the Committee on Science, Technology, and Law. He currently chairs the IOM Committee on National Preparation for Mass Disasters and has chaired committees on privacy, genomics, and prisoner research. The IOM awarded Prof. Gostin the Adam Yarmolinsky Medal for distinguished service in furthering its mission of science and health. He also received the Public Health Law Association's Distinguished Lifetime Achievement Award. Internationally, Prof. Gostin received the Rosemary Delbridge Memorial Award from the National Consumer Council (U.K.) and the Key to Tohoko University (Japan) for distinguished contributions to human rights in mental health.

Prof. Gostin has led major law reform initiatives in the United States, including the drafting of the Model Emergency Health Powers Act to combat bioterrorism and the "Turning Point" Model State Public Health Act. He is also leading a team developing a Model Public Health Law for WHO and drafting a Framework Convention on Human Services for The World Bank—a multilateral treaty on the health care professional capacity in poor and middle-income countries.

Maria Merritt, Ph.D., is a core faculty member of the Johns Hopkins Berman Institute of Bioethics and assistant professor in the Department of International Health (Health Systems Program) at the Johns Hopkins Bloomberg School of Public Health. She is a co–associate director of the Greenwall Fellowship Program in Bioethics and Health Policy and a faculty affiliate and advisory board member of the Johns Hopkins–Fogarty African Bioethics Training Program. Dr. Merritt holds a career development award (2009–2012) funded by the Greenwall Faculty Scholars Program in Bioethics. Her research interests include bioethics, global health ethics, international research ethics, moral philosophy, and moral psychology.